Nursing
Homes

Nursing
Homes

Too Old Too Sick Too Bad

Nursing Homes in America

Frank E. Moss, J.D.
former U.S. Senator

Val J. Halamandaris, J.D.

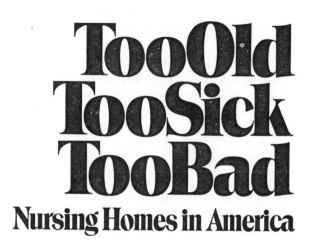

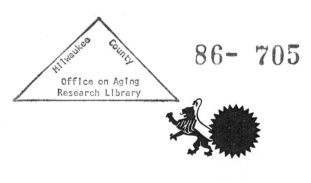

Aspen Systems Corporation
Germantown, Maryland
1977

Library of Congress Catalog Card Number: 77-72515
ISBN:0-912862-43-2

Printed in the United States of America.

3 4 5

*To our older Americans, who have helped
make this country great.*

Table of Contents

Acknowledgments

We gratefully acknowledge the assistance of so many who aided us in our study of nursing home problems. Among those who have been the most helpful are Senators Frank Church, Pete V. Domenici, Edward M. Kennedy, Lawton Chiles, and Sam Nunn, who have had an active interest in long term care. Congressman Claude Pepper, chairman of the House Committee on Aging, and his staff director, Robert Weiner, are also to be commended for their work in this field. The staff of the Senate Committee on Aging have played an important role in helping to bring the facts about nursing homes to light. Staff Director Bill Oriol and Chief Counsel Dave Affeldt have been especially helpful.

Others who have been of invaluable assistance through the years include: Nelson Cruickshank, president, and William R. Hutton, executive director of the National Council of Senior Citizens; Cyril Brickfield, counsel of the National Retired Teachers Association — American Association of Retired Persons; Larry Lane, government relations director, American Association of Homes for the Aged; Gus Johanson, supervisory auditor, U.S. General Accounting Office; Burt Seidman and Larry Smedly of the AFL-CIO; Charles J. Hynes, New York's special prosecutor for nursing homes; William D. Cabin, executive assistant to New York Secretary of State Mario M. Cuomo; Frank Frantz, long time expert in the field of long term care; Dr. Robert Butler, director of the National Institute on Aging; Elma Griesel and Chuck Chomet of the Citizens Coalition for Nursing Home Reform; and author Bill Halamandaris, who helped edit the manuscript.

Three people must be singled out for special thanks. Daphne Krause, executive director of the Minneapolis Age and Opportunity Center directs the best program of protective in-home services for the aged in the United States. Her program is a model of what should be duplicated all over America. She has extensive knowledge of the operations of nursing homes, and her efforts on behalf of senior citizens in the Twin Cities area have made her a legend. It was through Daphne Krause that we first met John Edie. John had the responsibility of investigating nursing home abuses for her in preparation for the Minnesota hearings conducted by our Subcommittee on Long Term Care. John's work was so impressive that the committee hired him to work in the national nursing home investigation. He left his mark on many of the hearings which were subsequently held, notably, the subcommittee's 1975 New York efforts. The 12-volume subcommittee report is evidence of his many abilities. We are grateful to John for all his help without which this book may never have been written. John left the committee staff on October 1, 1975 to become deputy director of the California Office on Aging.

Senator Charles Percy has served as ranking Republican on the Subcommittee on Long Term Care. He has attended every hearing and meeting. Together, we have conducted hearings in all parts of the country. He has demonstrated his personal commitment to nursing home reform not only by working to enact legislation, but by visiting nursing homes in Illinois almost every weekend. There is no one who has done more to advance the cause of the elderly than Senator Percy.

Preface

This book reflects an intensive 14-year effort to learn the truth about nursing homes. It began in 1963, when I first joined the Senate Committee on Aging. At that time it was apparent to me that with the ever-increasing number of older Americans, nursing homes would have growing importance. For this reason, I asked the members of the Senate Committee on Aging for permission to bring together our health and housing subcommittees to conduct an investigation into problems in the area of long term care. As chairman of the combined subcommittees, I presided over hearings which proved to be of such importance that the committee established a permanent Subcommittee on Long Term Care in 1965. I was named chairman of that subcommittee.

In 1965, we launched an eventful series of hearings across the nation, compiling about 1,300 pages of testimony. These hearings to some degree shaped the Medicare and Medicaid acts and resulted eventually in the enactment of a comprehensive series of reforms known as the Moss and Kennedy amendments of 1967. The failure of the Department of Health, Education, and Welfare first to implement these amendments with suitable administrative regulations, and later to enforce them, ranks as the great tragedy explored in this book.

HEW took until June of 1969 to offer the first proposed standards in implementation of the Moss amendments. Paradoxically, these amendments, as implemented by HEW, actually had the effect of lowering requirements for nursing homes participating in federal programs. In protest, I called the first in what was to become a series of 30 hearings between 1969 and 1976. As we began these hearings, I asked my long-time friend, Val J. Halamandaris, associate counsel with the Senate Committee on Aging, to direct an intensive investigation of nursing homes.

Val is responsible for the research and associated work of the Subcommittee on Long Term Care. He personally wrote the subcommittee's 12-volume report, "Nursing Home Care in the United States: Failure in Public Policy." He is more than a skilled and attentive attorney; his investigatory skills are rooted in concern and, where necessary, outrage. He has provided Congress with more insights and information on the nursing home industry than it has ever had before. In the past two years, Val has also directed our investigations into fraud and abuse among practitioners, clinical laboratories, and Medicaid mills. All of these efforts single him out as one of the nation's leading experts on the subjects of health, aging, and long term care.

After our eight years of work together, we were convinced that this book was necessary in order that the truth about nursing homes as we had learned it might reach the American public. This book is not an attempt to indict the entire nursing home profession. There are many fine homes in America whose very existence proves we need not tolerate poor care and abuse.

We describe the history of nursing homes in America and attempt to illustrate graphically what happens in nursing homes today. We attempt to show why it happens and what can be done about it. We have also made a special effort to help families who are faced with the difficult decision of how to choose a nursing home. At the same time, we offer this as a textbook to help administrators learn what they might do to improve the operation of their homes and to help erase the negative image associated with nursing homes. However, our first and overriding concern is the welfare of the millions of older Americans who suffer the compound burdens of illness and advanced age.

We hope that this book will lead to greater understanding and to increased pressure for reform.

Frank E. Moss
May 1977

Introduction

Not long ago a newspaper in the Midwest carried a classic story which describes what can happen when good men and women, regardless of their age or background, are pushed up against the wall of injustice:

Topeka. Kansas police were called today to help restore order at a Methodist home for the aged, scene of a week-long revolt. Three militant octogenarians were arrested after a scuffle in the north parlor. They were identified as leaders of an activist group that seized control of the parlor three days ago and locked Mrs. Norma Sunderland, charge nurse, into the closet.

George Whitlock, 84-year-old spokesman for the activists told a reporter the demonstration was staged to enforce demands that the old folks be given more role in management.

"We have a bunch of young whippersnappers running things around here," he said, waving his cane indignantly. "We don't trust anybody under 65," he added, proudly displaying his senility power button pinned to his shawl.

Two officers suffered minor injuries during the disturbance. One was hit by a runaway wheelchair and the other was jabbed by a knitting needle.

The revolt began last week when a small group of hardnosed superannuates held a dodder-in at which some burned their Social Security cards. Although peaceable in the early phases, the protest movement took on a violent turn when someone hit Emery Dains, home administrator, with a bottle of Geritol. Mr. Dains blamed the trouble on a misunderstanding caused by difficulties in communicating with the militants.

"Some turn off their hearing aids when administrative personnel seek to explain policies, etc.," he explained. Mr. Whitlock reacted, "What is the sense of living a long time if some kid who is only 45 to 50 years old can tell you what you have to do?"[1]

This account is amusing because it is well written, but it also is painfully relevant. It describes what can happen if the nation's infirm elderly resort to some of the tactics which have been used by other groups who feel bypassed these days. It also illustrates the point that for years nursing homes have been hidden away from the mainstream of society. Their exact role has been little understood. These facts are further demonstrated by the following examples.

Two young boys were talking on a street in Brooklyn, New York. One of them mentioned that his grandmother had been placed in a nursing home. "What's a nursing home?" asked the other young lad. "That's where they keep dead people they ain't buried yet," came the reply.

A similar conversation took place in a Florida home for the aged. Various senior citizens were expressing their views about nursing homes. "Nursing homes are the beginning of the end," said one old man. Another man countered with his actual experience in a Florida facility. According to him, patients were beaten, the food was inedible, and the quality of care was poor. "I was lucky to escape," he said. "I was one of the few who made it out." Asked to compare his experience in a nursing home with his imprisonment in a Nazi concentration camp, he answered, "Dachau was cleaner." A third old man had exhausted his savings taking care of his wife who had just died in a Michigan home. "Being in a nursing home is a lot like waking up in a coffin," he offered. "You say to yourself that if I am here, I am either dead or I soon will be."

This prevailing and highly negative view of nursing homes is shared by most people in America. To a large extent, this view has been reinforced by the news media. For example, the Associated Press recently published a detailed study of nursing homes and concluded:

Despite a billion dollar bonanza from the federal government, America's nursing homes are a stark lonely place to die.

Abuses in money and medicine, an air of death and despair shadow the aged through the dusk of their days.

Doctors rarely see patients. Nurses use drugs freely to restrain patients. Mental patients are placed into nursing homes by the thousands. And fraud feeds on the federal dollar.

While the prevailing public opinion about nursing homes is negative, in-depth interviews reveal that this is largely an emotional reaction. When pressed for an intellectual response, most people had difficulty defining a nursing home or outlining the services that it should offer. Most commented the institution was something like a small hospital but with no doctors.

Knowledgeable physicians who work with nursing home patients on a daily basis have still different views. In an article which appeared in the *Salt Lake City Tribune* April 16, 1972, Dr. Victor Kassel, world-famous Utah geriatrician and author, put it this way: "The aged are betrayed just as are the poor. Our continual neglect will partially solve the problem. The nursing homes will do our dirty work. We pay them inadequately to insure inferior care. The doctors abandon their patients to insure no medical follow-up. Behind closed doors we await gerocide. We expiate our guilt by pointing to the heartless nursing home administrator."

Dr. Naomi Bluestone provides this penetrating insight:

> I made the rounds of the nursing homes, where the sick elderly marinated in their own urine or slumped over the arms of that familiar paraplegic roost, the wheelchair. . . . I have learned that this is the way it is to be. I know now that the enemy may be cloaked in the coat of the healer, and that a friend will appear from the lowliest of our society. I have learned how the purse strings tighten a noose around our therapeutic efforts and force us to employ for our elderly those whom no one else will have, but they alone do not cause our travail. I have perceived that repression springs from a terrified heart, so untutored voices speak to us of euthanasia to try to right our multiple wrongs. A society which will not care for its mothers and fathers will care just as little for its useless children. Some day we will all be held accountable for what we have done to our parents.

Nursing home owners and administrators have their own view. They are resentful of having to care for what they term society's unwanted balast. They claim that the elderly and the media are overreacting; operators, they say, provide good care, especially given the inadequate amount they are paid. They assert that families complain because of heavy guilt feelings which arise from placing relatives in long term care facilities. They add that those who visit a nursing home are repelled by the natural human condition and not by the quality of care offered by the facility. J.I. Green, executive director of the Minnesota Nursing Home Association, put it this way: "It would probably be natural for me to want to attack those that have been garbage-mouthing our profession. . . . The charges have put a tainted label on the entire profession, a label that's totally unfair, untrue or unwarranted."

In the past 16 years the American public has increasingly been confronted with these conflicting views of nursing homes and the kind of care they offer. During this same period, the number of nursing homes in the United States has increased 140 percent to about 23,000 homes; 80 percent are operated for profit. Nursing home revenues increased 2,000 percent from $500 million in 1960 to $10.5 billion in 1976. This startling increase is largely the result of the enactment of Medicare and Medicaid, two programs under growing attack as being riddled with fraud and abuse. Nursing home fees today account for fully one-third of the monies paid out in the $15 billion Medicaid program.

This book is an effort to reconcile the conflicting opinions about this controversy, to bring the truth to the American public. It describes what happens in nursing homes, why it happens, and what can be done about it.

The importance of this topic should be obvious because, as James Michner observed, "The problem of caring for the aged looms as the principal social problem of the balance of the century: greater than ecological asphyxiation; greater than overpopulation; greater than the energy crisis."[2]

In more personal terms, if present trends continue, at least one out of five of us will spend some time in a nursing home. In fact, each of us — every American — will deal with nursing homes in one of several roles, if not as a patient, then as a family member or friend of a patient.

Val J. Halamandaris
Washington, D.C.
May 1977

"MOTHER, A MAN HERE TO ASK SOME QUESTIONS"

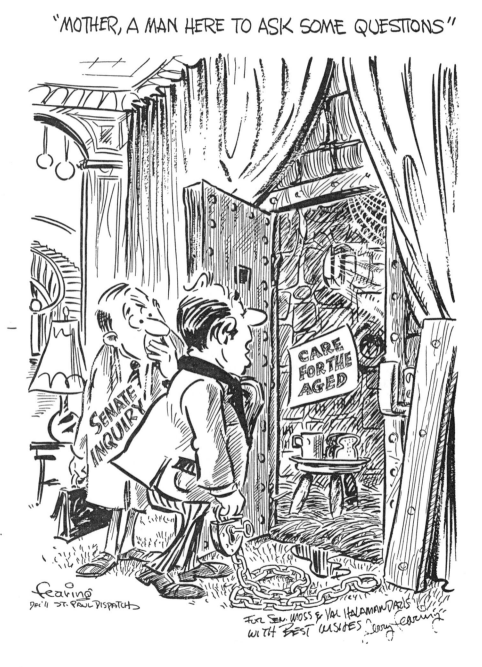

Part I
A Kaleidoscope of Nursing Home Problems

The eight chapters which make up Part I of this book are an attempt to describe accurately what happens in nursing homes. They answer the following questions: What are the most prevalent problems in nursing homes? Which are the most serious from the patients' point of view? Are nursing home abuses isolated instances or widespread industry practices? Do nursing homes deserve their negative image?

Chapter 1

Nursing Homes: The Greatest Fear of the Elderly

It's hell to be old in this country. This is a simple truth for most of our 21 million elderly. The pressures of living in the age of materialism and the pursuit of the good life have produced a youth cult in America. Our preoccupation with staying young knows virtually no boundary. We spend millions on elixers and remedies all the way from pep pills to hair transplants and face liftings. Hang the expense. Drink Pepsi, drive a Ford, smoke Silva Thins or do anything else anyone suggests might keep you looking young.

Why this obsession with youth? Some blame the movies. Others blame advertising for the images sold to the public. The real reason lies deeper. Most of us are afraid of growing old. This is true because we have made old age in this country a wasteland. It's T.S. Eliot's rats walking across cast-away bones. It's nowhere, in between this life and the great beyond. It's being robbed of your eyesight, your mobility, and even your human dignity.

It is evidence of our shameful and bankrupt policy toward the aged that one out of four of us can expect to live in poverty when we reach our 65th birthday. Most of us can expect less than half of the income we enjoyed when we were young. All of us will see the value of our savings and pensions greatly eroded by inflation. Those of us who want to work will have great difficulty finding a job; if we do land a job we will be allowed to earn only a miniscule amount before sacrificing some of our Social Security pensions.

If present trends continue, our medical bills will be three or four times as high at age 65 as they were when we were younger. It will likely cost us more and more out of pocket to participate in Medicare. And Medicare will cover less and less of our health bills. Today it only covers about 37 percent of the average senior citizen's health bill.

About 30 percent of us can expect to live in substandard housing without adequate plumbing or electricity. Those of us who do own our homes will have difficulty keeping them up. We will have more difficulty paying regressive real estate taxes which are already to the point of becoming confiscatory. Like the older American of today, we may suffer from physical isolation for the lack of transportation or from social isolation caused by separation from children, spouses, or other loved ones.

Taken together, these factors will produce social, emotional, and physical stress at the time when we are least able to deal with it. The collective impact may be damaging to personality. Confronted with these problems, some of us may try to "drop out" or may show little concern for life's events. Experts such as Dr. Victor Kassel, state unequivocally that these social problems can lead to increased organic illness:

> Too often during the past 17 years I have seen an elderly lady with arthritis return to an inadequate social environment at home with a hostile millieu. Upon arrival the patient becomes depressed and with depression further limitation in physical activity. Increased impairment from the arthritis results. This is a plain example of social pathology increasing organicity.

Other experts point to these problems as the reason that suicide rates between the years 55 and 84 are substantially higher than they are in the years prior to age 55.

Margaret Mead has pointed out what she believes to be yet another great disadvantage of America's policy toward the elderly—its effect on the younger members of society. She contends that society's present treatment of the elderly causes apathy or anxiety among the younger population and that it encourages a "live for now" attitude, or a lack of faith in the future.

All of these negative factors—age, despair and depression, poverty, physical and mental disability, and abandonment by society—exist to an even more startling degree with respect to the infirm elderly, especially those in nursing homes or other institutions. The infirm elderly suffer deep depression and have a comparatively reduced capacity for independent thought and action and low self-esteem.

Ralph Nader describes our treatment of the ill aged as "geriatric segregation," protecting society from the "curse and pestilence of age." He adds that nursing homes are the focus of all that has been wrought for old people in our society. Americans who have committed the crime of growing old and ill are exiled. They experience what psychiatrists call "social death" — the regression and death which Dr. Amos Johnson asserted is the natural result of this separation from the mainstream of society.

If it is hell to be old in America, it is something worse to be old and ill.

THE ORIGINS OF NURSING HOMES

The historical progenitors of nursing homes were almshouses, the public poor houses of colonial America. These facilities were the first American warehouses for the old and sick. They reflected the strict Puritan traditions of early America: poverty and illness were visible signs of punishment by a wrathful God.

The philosophy of isolating the aged and infirm from society continued to be the predominant social policy throughout the 18th and 19th century. A more charitable approach to the problem was late in developing. It was not until 1873 that the state of Connecticut established the first state board of charities.

The 20th century brought a phenomenal increase in the number of aged, resulting in changing social patterns. In 1900, there were about 3 million people in the U.S. over age 65, constituting four percent of the population. By 1975, their numbers had increased sevenfold to 21 million, or about ten percent of the total population. There are now 1.5 million people over 85, the fastest growing segment of our population. Life expectancy increased from 47 to 70 years during this same period.

There is no doubt that more and more people are living longer and longer. Modern medicine has saved those who previously would have succumbed to various diseases and disabilities. While mortality has been reduced, there has been a paradoxical increase in disability. This phenomenon has led some students of nursing homes wryly to observe that we have already turned Darwin on his head, i.e., that modern medicine perpetuates "survival of the unfittest." But there are other forces in operation which increase the likelihood of nursing home placement for today's golden-agers.

In years past, America was a more rural nation. This was the norm in the 19th century. The large influx of immigrants at the turn of the century is perhaps the benchmark in the transition of the U.S. from an agrarian to an industrial society. As the city became more and more the focus of American life, the traditional role of the elderly was undercut. In the city it becomes difficult to support three-generation families in which grandparents live with their children and grandchildren. The need to move from city to city to follow industrial employment and the mobility provided by the automobile have all had their part in the dissolution of the expanded family concept. Finally, Social Security has given the elderly their own funds and some measure of independence from their families. Many have preferred to live by themselves. Others have been cast adrift by their families with the rationale that the state has provided for them.

Ironically, it was the enactment of the Social Security Act of 1935 which created the unique for-profit system of nursing homes we have today. Social Security was an effort by Congress to provide some income security for the burgeoning numbers of aged. However, there was such a strong reaction at that time to conditions in public poor houses that Congress barred the payment of federal old age assistance funds to individuals housed in public institutions. The intent was to encourage the elderly to live at home or with foster families. The effect was the displacement of thousands from public facilities to privately owned for-profit boarding homes. In time, such facilities began to add nurses and to call themselves "nursing homes."

By the mid-1950s, the number of homes had grown substantially, and most states were licensing such facilities. Unquestionably, the greatest boost came in 1965 with the enactment of Medicare and Medicaid. Nursing homes changed from a family enterprise to big business. Major corporations, including several hotel/motel chains, purchased large numbers of facilities and nursing home issues became the hottest item on the stock exchange. Figure 1-1 illustrates the dramatic growth in the number of nursing homes, beds, and expenditures between 1960 and 1976. As noted, homes have increased 140 percent to 23,000. The number of nursing home beds has increased 302 percent to 1.3 million, outpacing general and surgical hospital beds by a good margin. Most dramatic is the 2,000 percent increase in revenues received by the industry. Almost $6 billion of the present $10.5 billion total is paid by the taxpayer through Medicare and Medicaid.[1] By contrast, the number of senior citizens increased 23 percent between these years.

Table 1-1 provides a profile of the more than one million patients in America's 23,000 nursing homes on any given day. As noted previously, this number is deceiving because studies indicate that one out of every five seniors will spend some time in a nursing home. It is obvious from a glance that most patients are women, very old, very sick, and

Figure 1-1 Estimated Gains in Number of U.S. Nursing Homes, Number of Beds, Employees and Expenditures for Care as Contrasted With the Increase in Number of Older Americans, by Percent (1960-1976)

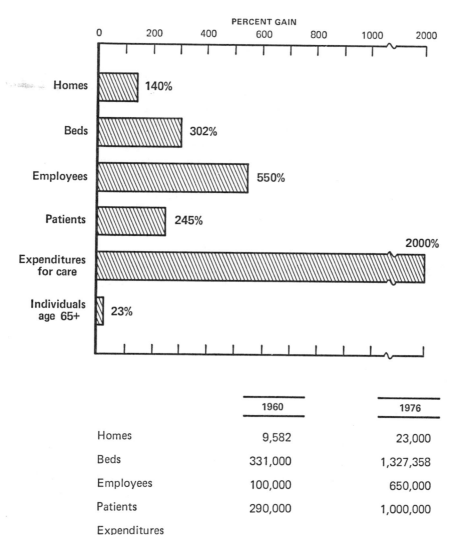

	1960	1976
Homes	9,582	23,000
Beds	331,000	1,327,358
Employees	100,000	650,000
Patients	290,000	1,000,000
Expenditures (millions)	$500	$10,500
Age 65-plus (millions)	17	21

very helpless. Unable to care for themselves, they must trust others for their protection.

Table 1-1 A Profile of America's One Million Nursing Home Patients

They are old:	Average age 82; 70% are over 70.
Most are female:	Women outnumber men 3 to 1.
Most are widowed:	Only 10% have a living spouse. Widowed, 63%; never married, 22%; divorced, 5%.
They are alone:	More than 50% have no close relatives.
They are white:	Whites, 96%; blacks, 2%; others 2%.
They come from home:	Some 31% came from hospitals, 13% from other nursing homes, the remainder from their own homes.
Length of stay:	An average of 2.4 years.
Few can walk:	Less than 50% are ambulatory.
They are disabled:	At least 55% are mentally impaired; 33% are incontinent.
They take many drugs:	Average 4.2 drugs each day.
Few have visitors:	More than 60% have no visitors at all.
Few will leave:	Only 20% will return home. Some will be transferred to hospitals, but the vast majority will die in the nursing home.

THE CATALOGUE OF FEARS

The phenomenon of large numbers of ill elderly is a comparatively recent development in the United States, as is the institution which has grown to meet the need. The solution (nursing homes) to this perplexing problem is typically American: turn it over to free enterprise. This solution also reflects the prevailing social policy of the times: the sick, the aged, and other nonproductive members of society are an embarrassment; they remind us of our own mortality and therefore should be removed from view.

It is little wonder then that our seniors regard nursing homes with trepidation. An analysis of this all-encompassing fear of nursing homes breaks down into several elements as described below. What all of them have in common is roots in contemporary attitudes toward aging and the aged.

The Fear of Being Old and Ill

Throughout recorded history, few fears have cut as deeply into the soul of man as the fear of growing old. The power of these fears is such that everyone has at some time prayed with the psalmist, "cast me not off in time of old age when my strength faileth." It is to cushion these fears that societies have adopted morality codes or laws which reflect the command, "Honor thy Father and thy Mother." The ancient Greeks, for example, enacted comprehensive legislation concerning care of the aged. Stiff penalties were exacted for violations. In ancient Athens, a Greek who neglected his parents could expect to be stripped of his most valuable possession — his citizenship. The laws and customs of other societies are summarized in Appendix A.

The historian Toynbee concluded that a society's quality and durability can best be measured by the respect and care it gives to its elderly citizens. Accepting this yardstick, very little can be said for either the quality or the durability of contemporary American society. As most seniors would be quick to agree, the United States, perhaps the richest nation in the world, is peculiarly bankrupt in its treatment of senior citizens.

In addition to fears generated by social policy, the aged have great fear of progressive physical and mental deterioration. To be old means being trapped in brittle bodies that respond rustily to the commands of a tired brain; it means having a memory that turns on and off like a neon sign. Every passing day increases the chances of illness or disability. To be old and ill is the worst of all. It is a time of no tomorrows, a time of no hope. Death lurks like a mugger in a dark alley. The elderly await the inevitable, when they are reduced to the simple act of breathing and eating — and less.

The Fear of Being Poor and a Burden

Almost all older Americans have fears associated with how they will be able to pay for the cost of a stay in a nursing home. Since the average nursing home costs about $800 a month and the average retired couple has about $400 in income, it is clear that few can afford to pay for the cost of care themselves. Those who make an effort to do so quickly use up whatever assets they might have. Many older Americans are afraid they will go broke, use up their savings, and lose their homes if they are sent to nursing homes. Moreover, they feel it will all be senseless since they have seen few nursing home patients restored. rehabilitated, and returned to the community.

The elderly know that after exhausting whatever funds they have on hand, the next step is to rely on their children and other relatives to assume their nursing home bills or go on welfare/Medicaid. For many senior citizens who embody the Puritan work ethic and who survived the Great Depression, going on welfare is a crime, the ultimate tragedy associated with worthlessness. Yet many take the pauper's oath to get care because they find it preferable to the alternative of becoming a burden on their families. Since the average nursing home patient is 82, it is clear that many may have children who are themselves aged. Those in the middle-aged bracket may well be supporting young children in college in addition to their aged parents. Regardless of age, the burden of an additional $800 per month would be an impossible load for most American families. The decision to place a loved one in a nursing home also places a heavy strain on the family structure. For the family, feelings of guilt, conflict, and shame may coexist with a subconscious desire to be relieved of a burden they have carried often beyond the point of toleration.

The Fear of Change and Uncertainty

Age brings with it too many shifting sands and not enough solid ground. The uncertainties of being placed in a nursing home take a significant toll on the elderly. Rigidity and resistance to change are endemic to age, and the shock all animals and plants experience when they are uprooted from their familiar environments is amplified in the elderly. Experts in the field of aging such as Elaine Brody, Ethel Shanas, and Margaret Blenkner have demonstrated the increases in mortality and morbidity that occur when people are institutionalized. In one study, Blenkner documented a 42 percent death rate among patients admitted to nursing homes as compared with 28 percent for similar individuals awaiting admission. This phenomenon has been termed transfer trauma or transplantation shock. To identify fully, one need only remember what it was like to be the new kid on the block or recall the anxiety associated with leaving home for the armed forces or a distant college.

The Fear of Insanity

Oscar Nelson is a case in point. This fastidious 75 year old lived alone but had the unhappy habit of forgetting to take his heart pills.

Relatives in a distant city placed him in an Ohio nursing home "for his own good." He was given a room by himself on the home's first floor — the home's show floor. Many prospective customers were shown Oscar's neat room as an example of the care the facility offered. Every day Oscar put on his pin-striped suit and enjoyed his daily walk to the corner grocery and to Kelley's Bar.

One day he saw an aide strike a patient and reported the incident to the state health department. In retribution, the administrator sent Oscar "to the zoo" — the home's third floor where all the incontinent, mentally imparied, and dying patients were kept. Oscar's two new roommates were the most hopelessly confused on the entire floor. One of them insisted Oscar was his "no good brother." At night, Oscar would wake from a sound sleep to find this giant standing over him with his hands about Oscar's throat.

Oscar's cries for help resulted in his being cited as a behavioral problem. Tranquilizers were administered. Within two weeks Oscar was babbling like everyone else. He sat for hours in his own waste, dressed only in a hospital gown — tied to the chair with the sleeves of a blue pin- striped jacket.

But, Oscar is not alone. In St. Paul, Minnesota, one patient jumped three stories to her death because the home gave her a roommate who spanked her fellow patients believing they were her babies, ran around with her dress up over her head, and drank from the toilet.

The fact is, the great majority of nursing home patients (55 to 80 percent) are mentally impaired, and the elderly realize that exposure to them along with other conditions may result in insanity. Simple behavior adaption would make it so.

Dr. Herbert Shore of Dallas, Texas, former president of the American Association of Homes for the Aging, has written about old people caught in the vicious spiral of senility. It begins with others' demanding that the old person abdicate accustomed roles in life, which decreases the sense of identity and self-worth, which in turn is followed by failing health and/or initial signs of brain damage. At this point, others insist that the aging person become dependent upon various institutions for care and protection. Institutionalization and the social stigma associated with it further decrease the sense of identity and self worth. The aged person reacts by becoming confused, docile, or uncooperative. The aged person then comes to accept as a fact this imposed sense of worthlessness, further retreating into the past and losing any meaningful concern for the unpalatable present. Consequently, the person is labeled unreachable or hopelessly senile. Vegetation and death follow directly.

The Fear of Losing Liberty, Identity, and Human Dignity

The New York Civil Liberties Union (NYCLU) has classed nursing homes with other total institutions which attempt to control every aspect, every personal detail of their clients' lives. "They virtually abolish privacy, stifle individuality, deify the values of order and discipline and enforce arbitrary and discretionary rules. Viewed as a polity, these institutions can only be described as totalitarian. And indeed, those unfortunates who are confined to such institutions have much in common with residents of a totalitarian political regime."

As the NYCLU points out, nursing home patients differ from prisoners and inmates in mental institutions. Residents of nursing homes have neither been declared incompetent nor convicted of a crime. Consequently, nursing home patients are entitled to enjoy the same rights guaranteed to the rest of us by the Constitution and the Bill of Rights.

It is paradoxical, then, that entry into a long term care facility invariably means a loss of rights, privileges, and prerogatives. Choices become fewer and fewer. The elderly find that they cannot do what they want to do when they want to do it. Most of all, they cannot go home. It is a regulated, regimented existence.

Nursing home operators justify the limitation of these freedoms, claiming the need for order throughout the home. They insist they do what they do in the best interests of all the residents. Some insist on infantilizing their patients or plying a heavy layer of paternalism.

To make matters worse, the aged fear a loss of identity when they are asked to leave behind the security of a familiar environment. Many homes forbid your taking with you all the little things that help remind you who you are. Left behind or soon lost are clothes, watches, jewelry, a cat, a favorite chair, faded photographs—all the benchmarks of a lifetime which tell you upon awakening in the morning that you are home and not in some Holiday Inn in Pittsburgh.

The loss of identity, freedom, and independence is a forced divestiture of human dignity and almost all aspects of self. Such total divestiture is what has been termed social death.

The Fear of Death

As has been implied many times, seniors fear nursing homes because of their intimate connection with death. It is to nursing homes that the elderly are sent in their final hours. Most of those who enter a nursing home will never come out alive. In fact, in one study, some 27 percent of those entering a nursing home died within the first month of their stay.

A survey conducted by the University of California indicated that nursing homes are the last place the elderly would choose even for death. Some 61 percent preferred to die at home, 31 percent at a hospital, and only 2 percent preferred dying in a nursing home.

The Fear of Poor Care and Abuse

Most senior citizens have visited nursing homes or talked with people who have. They understand that most patients are helpless and must rely on the assistance of nursing home personnel. The espoused goal of the caretakers is the three Rs: to restore, rehabilitate, and return to the community. But the fact that the elderly see so few of their friends restored, rehabilitated, or returned reinforces their negative image of nursing homes.

The news media also report seemingly endless negative stories about nursing home care. A Miami newspaper told of eleven elderly people rejected by their relatives and by nursing homes, abandoned in wheelchairs or stretchers in the emergency room of a Miami hospital with "Do Not Return" labels pinned to their clothes. The *Idaho Statesman* recently described that state's investigation into possible wrongdoing by an Idaho nursing home in a patient's death from unattended gangrene. The *Washington Post* reported the conviction of a nursing home operator and a nurse's aide on the charge of murdering a patient in a Washington, D.C. nursing home. In the days following July 27, 1970, the *Baltimore Sun* carried stories of an outbreak of salmonella which ultimately claimed 36 lives in a Baltimore nursing home.

In addition to reporting news events such as fatal fires and epidemics in nursing homes, the newspapers have conducted in-depth investigations. In the past ten years more than 60 have been published describing nursing homes as warehouses for the dying. They report endless examples of negligence, poor care, poor food, excessive use of drugs, profiteering, and unsanitary conditions.

In the end, senior citizens, like Will Rogers, believe what they read in the newspapers. They believe Ralph Nader, who charges that the chain of nursing home abuses are more epidemic than episodic. They agree with Florida's Thomas Routh in describing nursing homes as "a cross between an asylum and the Spanish inquisition, masquerading as the greatest boon ever given to an ungrateful segment of the population."

The average senior citizen looks at a nursing home as a human junkyard, as a prison, a kind of purgatory, halfway between society and the cemetery, or as the first step of an inevitable slide into oblivion. Nursing homes are not only synonymous with death, but with the notion of protracted suffering before death. It is clear that seniors view nursing homes through the dark glass of emotionalism and that there is a need for an objective review of the litany of nursing home abuses.

Chapter 2

Nursing Home Abuses

On a hilltop just outside of Pittsburgh, Pennsylvania, standing against the skyline like a fortress, is the J.J. Kane Hospital, the second largest nursing home in the United States. It is owned by Allegheny County and has been in operation for about 10 years. For its 2,200 beds and almost as many residents, it boasts a yearly $19 million budget, most of which is public Medicaid funds. In terms of county outlays, the nursing home accounts for more dollars than any other service. In fact, expenditures equal the total spent for parks and recreation, courts and jails, police and fire training combined.

The facts revealed during the Senate subcommittee's investigation of Kane Hospital provide great insight into the kinds and dimensions of nursing home abuses. Following the Kane Hospital narration are selected examples of abuse which the subcommittee has documented. Collected from various facilities across the nation, these generic examples are a mirror image of what is happening in nursing homes and give some indication of how widespread these problems are.

KANE

Two male aides were struggling to pull a young, multiple sclerosis patient out of bed into a wheelchair for an infrequent bath. "I'll take care of him myself," said one aide slammming the patient into the chair. The patient groaned. The aide smiled at the patient and said, "You know I hate Dagos, don't you?" The patient was taken to a bathtub and sat quietly as the aide continued to berate him. "You know I hate you. Now that you are in the tub, I ought to drown you." The aide soaked a washcloth in the water and slapped the patient on the head and shoulders with it several times. "The headline in tomorrow morning's paper is going to read, 'Aide Kills Patient in Bathtub', you Dago son of a bitch . . .'" and slapped the patient with a wet washcloth again. This time the patient grabbed hold of the cloth. The aide punched him in the arm, forcing him to let go of the cloth, and decided that the bath was finished. The man, not wanting to be dropped, stiffened up as the aide lifted him out of the tub. He was punched in the stomach, pushed back in a wheelchair, hastily dried, and returned to his room.

The aide returned with another wheelchair patient to bathe. This was a black man, in his 70s and unable to walk. While undressing him for the bath, the aide discovered that the patient had a mild case of diarrhea. The aide lifted the man into the the empty tub and began to spray him in the face with cold water from the sprayer used to clean out the tub after baths. The man cried out, begging him to stop. The aide told him, "You better learn never to shit yourself again, nigger," and sprayed the man with cold water again. "Hey, watch him jump," said the aide to a colleague. He adjusted the sprayer so that a forceful half-inch jet of cold water came out, turned it on full, and sprayed the man's genitals. The patient screamed and covered his genitals with his hands. The aide whispered, "Do you know why I hate you? . . . cause you're a nigger."

Holding the man's hands, the aide sprayed him again with cold water, this time the sprayer less than a foot away from the man's genitals. The aide then interrogated the man. "Are you a black man?" The patient did not respond. The aide (louder), "Are you a black man?"

"Yes," said the patient softly.

"Are you a nigger?" The patient did not reply. "Are you a nigger'?" demanded the aide in a loud voice.

"Yes."

"Is this nigger ever going to shit again?"

"No," responded the patient weakly.

The preceding lines read something like a Dickens novel, but they are, in fact, verbatim testimony presented to the Subcommittee on Long Term Care by present and past employees of Kane Hospital. They contacted the subcommittee in June of 1975, having been directed there by a senior citizens activist group, the Gray Panthers, located in Philadelphia.

Former employees Joseph Nagy and Mary Lewin told of their early efforts to reform Kane Hospital from within and how they were rebuffed by the administration. They spoke of their determination to bring about change by compiling a record of events and releasing it to the press. They presented the subcommittee with a draft of their report which contained the above incidents and a host of other charges.

They charged that the county commissioners (who were in office at the time) were using the hospital's service contracts and its 1,800 jobs as political patronage and that favored employees were not required to attend work regularly. The hospital misled the public, they added, through a large public relations budget. All employees were threatened with the loss of their jobs if they were not "loyal to the hospital."

They provided evidence that the facility falsely declared patients in need of skilled nursing care (and thus qualifying them for the highest rate of Medicaid reimbursement) even though the patients needed only custodial care. Evidence was offered that patients were admitted because of political pressure and that they were retained for similar reasons after they had recovered. In one case, a social worker's efforts to discharge a patient met with an irate family, the intervention of a state senator, and direct orders from the director to leave the patient alone.

The employees spoke of physicians' inattention, pointing out that in many areas of Kane, doctors' notes and medication orders were prewritten by nurses and falsified in order to pass government inspection. Although hospital regulations require that patients be seen by physicians at least once a day, one man said he had not seen a doctor in more than a year and a half. Asked about the examination, he described the elderly practitioner and quipped, "He needed a doctor about as bad as I did." In his statement to Nagy, the man remembered that the examination consisted only of two or three questions such as "How old are you?"

Kane Hospital was also described as being continually short of staff. Despite a state standard of 2.5 hours of nursing time per patient per day, Kane provided only 1.5 hours a day. Because of a shortage of basins, sheets, laundry, bedpans, urinals, and catheter plugs, a number of shortcuts were taken. "Mouth care was unheard of as was the sterilization of bedpans." Catheters were reused. Bathing patients was backbreaking work because of the lack of mechanical assitance. It was easier to give patients a sponge bath or to roll their wheelchairs into the shower and turn on the water.

There was little respect for patients' privacy. Patients were "actively discouraged from wearing their own clothes." Much of this personal clothing was never returned from the laundry; it was "lost" or went to another floor. Men wore either green pajama pants and tops or the familiar hospital gown. Women, who were given only the short hospital gowns, complained that their genitals were exposed when seated.

Many areas did not have draw curtains over beds. Perhaps most offensive was the procedure for changing patients who were wet or covered with bowel movements. One Kane employee described the procedure:

> First, we push all the patients in geri-chairs or wheelchairs back into an aisle in the ward, and then screen off the door. We wet a lot of towels and leave them in the sink. We work from one end of the line to the other. There is no privacy when this is going on—everybody sees each other. Some of the aides handle patients roughly—slapping, arm twisting and jerking goes on. Every day the patients get sworn at—asked if they are 'full of shit today' and called 'old bastards' and the like. Some patients fight back during changes, but most are scared and offer no resistance. The patient's restraints are untied and his gown is unsnapped and removed. Then the aide in front pulls the patient by his arms to a standing position naked, and holds him there, while the other aide wipes his buttocks with a wet towel from the sink and puts a clean pad on his chair. The patient is then dropped back into his chair and a new gown is slipped over his arms and snapped behind his neck. No effort was usually made to clean and dry patients who had urinated.

In some cases, patients were "padded" with 3 or 4 folded sheets under their buttocks instead of being given a bedpan when necessary. The sheets were pulled out one after another when the patient wet the bed. Such padding is prohibted even by Kane's rules because it quickly leads to bedsores. In some cases catheters were installed when unnecessary; it was done for the convenience of the staff. This practice leads to the loss of bladder tone and then to permanent incontinence.

The facility was seriously faulted for its poor handling of infectious diseases. Infected patients were generally permitted to remain in their own rooms; they were never provided with separate toilet and bathing facilities. This, coupled with the serious lack of clean linen, created "an imminent health hazard" in the opinion of the former employees.

Despite Pennsylvania law, which limits distribution of drugs to licensed practical and registered nurses, unlicensed aides at Kane distributed medications. In some cases, doctors signed medications orders without seeing the patient. "Often the medication for the whole floor (48 patients) would be ordered without the doctor seeing a single patient." One nurse added, "The way that medication is passed out around here is chaotic. No general hospital would stand for it." Similarly, patients were given tranquilizers — not out of need, but to make it easier on the staff.

Lewin and Nagy charged that patients were placed in restraints for the same reason. In fact, about one-fourth (500) of the patients were confined to geriatric chairs for a full day:

> A lot of people on my floor are tied with restraints in geri-chairs. Geri-chairs are like the high chairs babies eat in, except they are for adults. They have foot rests and trays that clamp around a person. Once someone is clamped in, they can't move around or get out. Geri-chairs have rollers wheels so the nurses aides can move people to where they want them. About one-quarter of the people at Kane Hospital are confined in geri-chairs all day long. People who have difficulty walking or are troublemakers, are kept in geri-chairs. They are lined up in hallways, against walls and around tables. Often they stay in one place all day long. Often the staff doesn't have time for regular bathroom trips with all the people on the floor, so geri-chairs patients sit in wet and dirty clothing.

This charge is all the more serious in view of the strict Pennsylvania law which limits the use of restraints to situations in which everything else has been tried and the patient continues to be a danger to himself or to others. Under such circumstances, a physician can order restraints, but even then the order must be in writing and for a limited period.

With such a high percentage of patients in geriatric chairs, it should be no surprise that there was little restorative nursing or therapy at the home. It is stark testimony that "five times as many bodies leave the Kane morgue as the discharge office." The average stay of patients is about two years, and "although the express purpose of Kane is to rehabilitate patients, less than 200 patients are discharged every year. In the same period over 1,000 Kane residents die."

In yet another sad turn of events, those patients who were lucid and spoke out against the poor care and abuse were the subjects of reprisals. Nagy and Lewin provided examples of patients who were not fed or cleaned or were sent to less desirable areas of the hospital. They referred to the common practice of ordering psychiatric evaluations as a form of harassment. A report on one such examination ordered on a patient whose only problem was the she "demanded too much attention" reads:

> Reason for requesting consult: Patient refused to leave bed. This 83 year old female has many physical complaints including headaches and dizziness. She is said to be extremely negativistic and relatively uncooperative. She had cataract surgery but remains 'legally blind'. Mental status revealed an elderly woman in no acute distress....She was oriented in all spheres....Relatively little memory impairment....There was minimal paranoid ideation and depression. Would suggest she be pushed to comply with ward regulations. If this is unsuccessful would feel this patient is commitable.

They described the fate of another patient who demanded better care:

> Dorothy had Parkinson's Disease and diabetes. She said she couldn't move any part of her body except her mouth and eyelids. She was the most demanding patient on the floor. She would always ask for things she needed. She was screamed at, slapped and told to 'shut up' many times by the staff. I was told 'she made herself like this, she could walk if she wanted to—she could when she came onto the floor. Don't feed her, she can do it herself.' So tray after tray sat in front of her and was taken away untouched. She begged us not to bring the trays in. Eventually we got orders to feed her, so we did. Some of the aides fed her quickly with giant spoonfuls. When she began choking, they would take the tray away and tell her she was done. When her decubiti got really bad, she was put on a circolectric bed. She was afraid of the bed—afraid of her catheter being pulled out, of slipping, of getting her feet hurt and of getting hit on the head when we put her onto the litter. Some of the aides would play with the buttons on the bed when she was being turned. Make it rock. Put her head lower, keep her upright for a while so 'she wouldn't forget how to stand up.' She was afraid of baths. She was stiff and uncomfortable in the tub. She yelled about it. Some of the aides teased her and poured water in face. When she was put back in bed after the bath, she was thrown in roughly. She died on my day off. When I came in the aides talked about

how the floor would be much easier, because a walking patient had been sent in her place.

Employees, too, soon get the message. A social worker made the mistake of taking sides with a family who complained that their mother's possessions had been stolen by a particular aide. She volunteered that other families had reported similar problems with this aide. Consequently, the family pressed its complaint with the nursing home director, who informed the social worker "she had been wrong in saying anything—that her loyalty to the institution was in question and that she would face losing her job for what she had done."

A registered nurse with a background in hospital work pushed the staff to provide good care, but her efforts went unappreciated. Fewer and fewer people were assigned to her work area. "I was told to ease up. I've learned to keep my mouth shut about what goes on here."

It became increasingly clear that in addition to many hard-working, well-intentioned employees, Kane Hospital also had its share of sadists such as the orderly described in the beginning of this chapter. Nagy offers this episode as further proof:

> On my first day on the floor Sharon and Bonnie gave me a show. Two patients, Jo Parkings and Bessie Blake, were put next to each other in geri-chairs. Sharon got a sheet and covered herself like a halloween ghost and squatted behind the chairs. She grabbed Josephine's hand and hit Bessie with it. Both of them got frightened and yelled. Sharon hit Bessie on the side of the head and hit her with Josephine's hand again. Bonnie told Josephine to stop it and Sharon kept it up. The two patients began scratching, hitting and yelling at each other. Sharon uncovered herself and asked them what the matter was. Sharon covered herself again. This time when the fight was going she took the sheet and covered both of them with it. They began yelling so loud that Sharon was afraid the nurse would hear. She took the sheet off and separated the chairs.

According to the former Kane employees, many of these same individuals made a common practice of taking the best food from patients' trays and eating it themselves—not that the food was all that great to begin with. Reportedly the menu was repetitive and unimaginative. The quality was fair to poor, and quantities were small. Those in need of special diets were served the same as everyone else.

While these allegations of poor food and abuse were shocking, allegations of misuse of patient's funds were equally alarming. Nagy and Lewin charged that the hospital did not supply families with clear, itemized bills, that it charged Medicaid patients or their families over and above what was paid by Medicaid, that patients' funds were mingled with hospital operating revenues, and that funds belonging to dead or discharged patients were kept by the facility.

Perhaps most offensive of all was the nursing home's version of the "company store." By federal law, Medicaid patients are allowed to keep $25 a month from their Social Security as a personal spending allowance; if they have no Social Security, they receive a $25 subsidy from the government. At Kane not everyone received this allotment. Those who did, received it in the form of storebook coupons (in script). The patient could use this script to buy sandwiches and cigarettes at the Kane snack bar. Unfortunately, "snack bar prices are high—equal to or higher than prices at the local snack bar or store outside the hospital."

The profits from the storebook snack bar sales were used to support the meager entertainment offered at the facility. "Kane residents end up paying for the recreational activities provided at the hospital out of their own monthly personal allotment." Since script was issued, the $25 per patient per month in cash can be deposited accruing interest "which has never been turned over to patients, families or beneficiaries."

But the use of storebook coupons takes on yet another dimension. The employees reported that payment in the form of coupons, cash, or cigarettes was common in one-third of the areas of the nursing home:

> On floors where tipping is common, patients simply understand that they must pay for what they get. On days when few staff are working—patients offer a "tip," wink and say "don't forget about me later." Many patients "tip" unwillingly, knowing that only if they become floor favorites will their life at Kane Hospital be bearable. If a patient is not on the "good side" of the staff, it means no bath or shave, fewer clean clothes and linen, no socks, no help going to and from the bathroom, and sitting in urine and BM longer.
>
> One day, I went into the bathroom and found two women trying to help each other go to the bathroom. One could not walk, the other could walk only with support. Both were soiled with BM. Neither had been wiped recently. I got help from another aide. We got gowns and got the woman who

could walk cleaned up first. When she left we cleaned up the other woman. She offered us three dollars from her storebook. She said to come around to her bed in the afternoon and she would have it ready for us. We refused the tip. She started crying and apologized for making a mess for such nice people. She cried and cried. She said we would go to heaven if she had anything to do about it.

After reading this summary, it should be easy to reconstruct the shock, the dismay, and concern felt by the subcommittee staff. The immediate question was, "Can things really be that bad?" Senator Moss requested Val Halamandaris to conduct a detailed investigation to test the validity of these charges prior to holding a Senate hearing, and to learn if a Senate hearing would be necessary.

During the months of September, October, and November, 1975, Val Halamandaris and other staff members made 19 unannounced visits to the facility at different times of the day and night. The staff members talked with present and past employees and soon confirmed the validity of a great number of the charges made by Lewin and Nagy in their draft report.

On December 1, 1975, the full team of investigators returned for yet another visit accompanied by Dr. Robert Butler, now director of the National Institute on Aging and recent recipient of the Pulitzer Prize for his book, *Why Survive: Growing Old in America*, Margaret Cushman, RN, a consultant to the Committee on Aging from Yale University, also accompanied the investigators.

After this visit and a consultation with the officers and directors of Kane Hospital, it was the consensus of opinion that a Senate hearing was warranted. The director of Kane and the county commissioners were so notified on that day. A formal letter was sent thereafter by Senator Moss inviting them to attend and outlining the basic charges.

At the December 9, 1975 hearing William C. Cobbs, president of the Action Coalition of Elders, a Pittsburgh senior citizens group, appeared and presented the subcommittee with the final draft of the report, now entitled, "Kane Hospital: A Place to Die." Also testifying were former employees Nagy, Lewin, and Emily Eckel, along with present employees Father Hugh C. McCormley, chaplain at Kane, and Registered Nurses Joan Keifer and Eileen Frenchick. The hearing was summed up in one question, when Senator Charles Percy asked Father

McCormley, "Would you put your mother in Kane Hospital?" He
answered:

> Before I answer that, I would like to give a little background
> information. My mother is an invalid. She had a stroke 4 years
> ago, and we have been able to maintain her at home. At pres-
> ent, however, we are just running on a shoestring in our
> situation. We are inches away from making a decision. At
> times, we felt compelled to make the decision to put her in an
> institution. The only thing I can say is that I would rather
> bury my mother than ever put her in an institution, especially
> Kane.

One week after the Senate hearings, the Pennsylvania Department
of Health released an interim report which confirmed the evidence of
poor care and abuse at Kane. A full investigation was ordered leading
to an 85-page report issued June 17, 1976. That report corroborated in
detail the findings presented to the Senate committee. The facility's
license was suspended; it was given six months to come into compliance. The newly elected county commissioners ordered a far-
reaching administrative overhaul.

Meanwhile, in May of 1977, the General Accounting Office completed its audit of the financial affairs of Kane, as requested by
Senator Moss. The audit confirmed widescale mismanagement of patients' funds, requiring families to supplement Medicaid payments,
and double billing Medicare and Medicaid to the tune of half a million
dollars. The facility promised to make appropriate corrections.

A COMPENDIUM OF ABUSE

With this glimpse of the dimensions of abuse possible in one home, it
is now appropriate to survey the range of the problems most commonly found in American nursing homes. Almost all nursing homes
have at least one of these problems; some (Kane) have all of them; the
vast majority fall somewhere in between. Some of the instances
described took place in 1976, others a few years before. However, examples were carefully chosen and were not used unless the principle il-
lustrated is still valid today. The recurrence and continuity of abuses
over many years is in itself significant.[1]

Negligence Leading to Injury and Death

Negligence is conduct which is careless; it is a breach of duty which results in injury or a violation of a person's rights. Under the law, those injured by such wrongful conduct may sue and collect damages from those who cause such injury. Negligence on the part of nursing home personnel can have dire consequences:

- In California, someone left a container of Liquid Drano sitting next to a patient's bed. The patient drank it but did not receive medical attention for several hours. When she was taken to the hospital, eight hours later, emergency surgery was performed. She died about a week later from suffocation by ulceration and edema of the larynx.

- A woman's foot went unattended in another Chicago nursing home. Despite her daughter's repeated pleas for staff attention to her mother, she watched her mother's foot blacken and develop gangrene. It was finally amputated.

- A patient left unattended in a Chicago nursing home was allowed to drink and smoke. She fell asleep, spilling liquor in her lap, and then dropped a lit cigarette. She became a human torch.

- A woman complained to the New York Health Department that her mother, who suffered from paralysis, was scalded by an aide trying to give her a bath. The patient died within a week.

Deliberate Physical Injury

The responsibility of the nursing home for injuries caused to patients is not limited to acts of negligence. The home is also liable for deliberate or intentional conduct causing injury to another.

In January 1972, a nursing home administrator and a nurse's aide in a Washington, D.C. nursing home were charged and later convicted of murder. The apparent motive was that the administrator had forged the deceased's name in cashing one or more civil service retirement checks. The patient knew this and threatened to make trouble.

A witness from Iowa testified:

Our program has been responsible for closing up some of these nursing and custodial homes. One instance—where these people had been beaten by laths taken from the side of a home, where plaster has been put over it—I know; and can testify to this, definitely, that it is true. I have seen the lath marks on the bodies of 80-year-old women.

I know that these people go hungry. I know that they lie there day after day in their own filth. I know that they have their mouths taped shut with adhesive tape—because they dared to ask for a bedpan at 2 o'clock in the afternoon, while the aides played cards.

The Illinois Department of Health files report that:

A female patient age 93, totally blind, and with severe cardiac problems, was put into a chair with restraints despite doctor's orders that she should be in bed. The day after she entered the nursing home, an attendant struck her in the face with her fist to punish her for spilling a cup of water. Her attending physician called the woman's daughters and had them remove her from the home. She was transferred to her home and died a week later.

Unsanitary Conditions

Unsanitary conditions can be extremely dangerous. They may spread a virulent infection, as in cases presented to the subcommittee where food handlers did not follow proper hygienic procedures, where kitchen preparation equipment was left uncleaned, or where food was left out in the open at room temperature prior to being served. Perhaps the most tragic example of probable food poisoning was the 1970 Baltimore salmonella epidemic, which claimed 36 lives. The suspected cause was shrimp and deviled eggs left sitting at room temperature. In a similar circumstance, 30 patients died in an influenza epidemic in a St. Petersburg, Forida nursing home. Dr. George Dame, director of the Pinellas County Health Department, stated that during the week of March 14, 1976 state inspectors found inadequate inspection controls. Other examples of this problem include the following:

A nursing home patient appearing at the subcommittee's Minnesota hearings testified:

The bathroom condition in the nursing home was filthy. I had to walk with my bandaged foot in urine on the floors of the bathroom. I had the janitor bring me a bunch of clean rags, which I hid under my mattress. Then I would take two or three rags with me when I went to the bathroom. I didn't have very good balance, so when I got there I would drop one rag on the wet places and try to mop up the mess with the legs of my walker. I was not able to bend over very well to do this. Then I would use another rag to put down by the toilet to put my feet on. They were wrapped in gauze you know. The third rag I used, after wetting it, to wipe up the toilet seat that many times was full of feces.

An employee in a South Dakota nursing home wrote to the subcommittee:

I have witnessed and been a party to unsterile, unclean techniques in handling medications, dressings and laundry. I have witnessed techniques of self care among the staff possibly responsible for the spread of infections among the patients. These include aides serving breakfast, lunch, and dinner (in addition to their personal care functions) instead of food handlers; aides and orderlies being responsible for laundry at night.

The chief dietician of Cook County, Illinois testified concerning "one of the worst homes in the county:"

On that visit I found that the home was filthy and there was fecal material on the stairs. They were carrying the laundry right through the kitchen at serving time and the food and the laundry were in full sight of each other.

In 1970, the Detroit Health Department reported that a dead body was allegedly kept for two days near the center's food handling area, that fecal matter was found in a patient's bureau drawer, and that patients were allowed to sit in bed in their own waste.

Poor Food and Poor Preparation

Food is more than sustenance for nursing home patients; it is a happening, the major event of the day. Some nursing homes offer excellent meals, but many do not. The complaints received ran the gamut from watery soup and small portions all the way to unwholesome food. More often than not, homes serve poor food to save money.

Through its subpoena power, the subcommittee learned that one administrator spent 54 cents per patient per day for food while jails in Chicago spend 64 cents a day. Data supplied by the General Accounting Office (GAO) concerning 90 nursing homes in Tennessee, Colorado, and Massachusetts revealed that 22 of the homes surveyed (or 24 percent) spent less than $1 per patient per day in 1971. Only one home in each of the three states (3 percent) spent more than $2 a day for food. One home reported 37 cents per patient per day in 1969, 40 cents in 1970, 37 cents in 1971, and 52 cents in 1973.

There were examples of injuries induced by aides trying to feed individuals who had suffered some paralysis and of patients literally starving to death because they could not swallow. There were examples of patients who had choked to death when served hard-to-chew foods such as beef bacon. There were examples of patients not receiving special diets ordered by physicians, a violation of federal standards. Diabetics, for example, were served pancakes with regular syrup or the same meal, minus dessert, as other patients.

At the subcommittee's Chicago hearings, Chief Investigator Bill Recktenwald of the Chicago Better Government Association testified that he served 37 patients his first day of work in a local nursing home:

> The dinner consisted of a very small portion of lettuce with some type of dressing, a small portion of applesauce, a cup of coffee, one toasted cheese sandwich and a small bowl of soup. Each patient received some milk. On occasion the food ... was taken from one patient's plate by the help (that worked for you) and moved over to another person's plate to use up, to fill that plate or put the portion on it and sometimes it was moved even a third time.

An orderly at the Minnesota hearing testified:

> Sometime around the middle of September the home served hot oatmeal for breakfast. There were worms in the oatmeal. This was not the first time that worms had been found in the food. It usually happens on an off during the summer. On this particular day in September I had passed out all of the trays to the people who could feed themselves. When I got the tray for one of the male patients that I fed, I put the sugar on his cereal and started to get a spoonful when I noticed something

black in the oatmeal. I looked at it closer and found out that is was a black bug. I looked more carefully through the cereal and I found a lot of bugs in it. I found some smaller white bugs with black heads. I immediately went down and reported this to the kitchen. We tried to get as much of the oatmeal away from the patients as we could, but many of them had already eaten it. The cook told me that she had taken the meal from an open box that was kept in the kitchen area. One time they made Kool-aid with soap in it. One thing that I forgot to mention about the bugs in the cereal was that when the head nurse, Miss B., found out about it, she said to feed it to them anyway.

Misappropriation and Theft

Theft and misappropriation are quite common in nursing homes, according to complaints received by the subcommittee. Almost anything can be stolen: electric razors, clothes, jewelry, liquor, drugs, radios, or televisions. There is evidence strongly suggesting that many patients are not receiving welfare allotment designated as personal spending money. Property of the nursing home, including food and equipment, is sometimes stolen. Sometimes, patients themselves misplace certain items.

The 1972 Maryland Governor's Commission on Nursing Home Problems charged in its report that there was little consistency in handling personal spending money. Dean Daniel Thurz of the University of Maryland stated:

> Money is being accumulated that belongs to the patients without the patients being able to spend the money ... it is a scandalous situation and a major violation of the rights of the individual.

A nurse's aide offered this sworn statement:

> Often they will leave the home without their teeth, without their rings, watches and without any personal effects which they had come in with. One patient bought a brand-new suit because he knew he was going to die before too long. When he died he left the home without that suit. It was never found .....
> Employees regularly take food and groceries from the home.

An RN testified:

> Of the welfare money allotted to the patients, they are
> allowed to keep $2 with them on the floor. Any more than that
> is kept in the office. If they go to the hairdresser, the transac-
> tion is then carried through the business office. However,
> there was a woman who received $5 for a Mother's Day pres-
> ent. They talked her into putting the money in the office. She
> agreed and was assured that she could get the money any
> time she wanted. When she wanted to send it to a grandson,
> someone went down to get it and they were told that the $5
> had been taken because the husband owed the nursing home
> $25. Now he owed them only $20.

Inadequate Control of Drugs

The lack of control of drugs is one of the most critical and far-
reaching problems confronting the nursing home industry. Some experts suggested that 60 percent of the patients in nursing homes have
inadequate pharmaceutical services. In order to present this problem
in perspective, a full chapter of this book is devoted to the subject. At
this point, the November 1975 findings of the Kansas attorney general
in his investigation of nursing homes may give some brief indication of
the dimension of the problem.

> Every home was in violation of basic regulations relating to
> the storage and dispensing of narcotics and drugs. Every
> home was in violation of the basic regulations relating to the
> compilation of drug records.

> In every home, it was patently obvious that nonlicensed,
> unqualified personnel, even residents themselves could attain
> access to drugs and narcotics. We found that pill counts were
> not made. Records that were kept did not correlate with
> records of dispensing of drugs.

> Clear evidence of drug borrowing by nurses dispensing
> drugs was found. That is borrowing from one resident to give
> another for whom it was not prescribed. Retention of drugs
> prescribed for deceased residents was evidenced. In one
> home, the controlling interest was owned by the pharmacist

shown to be the only pharmacist filling prescriptions in that home as well as in two other homes in the community.

We found direct evidence that drugs were being prescribed by a doctor but were not dispensed.

We found outdated drugs. We found drugs not dispensed according to the schedule and at intervals prescribed by the doctor. In some cases, drugs were dispensed 2 or 3 hours off the prescribed dosage schedule.

Medicine vials were found to be used and reused without sterilization. Commingled drugs were found; some drugs prescribed for one patient were found on a shelf nearest the resident's roommate.

Other Hazards to Life and Limb

Many other hazards exist in nursing homes. Perhaps the greatest is the possibility of death by fire. (This problem is examined in Chapter 4.) Other hazards are caused by poor housekeeping and maintenance, which expose patients to infectious diseases. Some homes house patients in basements or attics, in violation of law and regulations.

In August of 1976, five people were found dead in a Boynton Beach, Florida nursing home. Investigations revealed that the air conditioning was habitually broken down. The deaths followed a heat wave that had pushed temperatures up into the 90s. An inspection for the period January 1 to May 19, 1976 indicated 84 incidents or violations of standards in the facility.

A patient in a Utah nursing home contracted lice. After the matter was reported to the health department, the nursing home quarantined her room. The only contact the patient was allowed was with aides treating her or serving meals. The patient felt disgraced and became mentally unstable. As a last resort, the home shaved the patient's head. Unable to cope with the protracted and unsuccessful treatment, she became completely withdrawn.

A nurse's aide in a Minnesota home testified:

One day we found out from Mrs. Bunn that another patient had died of tuberculosis. The Administration never told any of us about this patient dying of tuberculosis. We didn't find out until two weeks later and that was by accident. We double checked with one of the nurses on duty, and she confirmed it that Mr. A had died of tuberculosis. They never told us anything about it, and we had worked very closely with this patient, brushing his teeth for him and everything. There were also other patients that were in the same room with him before he went to the hospital.

Unauthorized or Improper Use of Restraints

The subcommittee has received many complaints about the use of restraints. A restraint is any technique, device, or drug which interferes with the free movement of a person and which cannot be easily removed by that person. According to the *Nursing Home Law Manual* published by the Health Law Center, Aspen Systems Corporation, restraints may be categorized as follows:

1. mechanical—an apparatus or device such as straps, straight jackets, or handcuffs;
2. manual—the use of attendants to grasp or hold a patient;
3. seclusion— physical separation from others, including isolation;
4. hydrotherapy—water treatment, which usually involves hot or cold baths (continuous or not), wet sheets, or cold packs; and
5. chemical—drugs and sedatives to stimulate or suppress motor functions.

All of the types of restraints mentioned above have been used in nursing homes. Almost all states require a physician's order before an individual can be restrained. Most state laws prohibit the use of some types of restraints, and most require careful monitoring of patients. For example, Arizona, Idaho, Indiana, Pennsylvania, and Wisconsin require that restrained patients be checked every hour. Maine requires supervision every half hour. Alabama, Delaware, Illinois, Maryland, New Jersey, and Tennessee limit the use of restraints to 24 hours—a physician must review and revalidate restraint orders each day. Minnesota requires that a special attendant be on duty on each floor where a patient is restrained.

Complaints about the use of physical restraints are fewer now than in previous years—perhaps because administrators feel that the use of drugs is a more appropriate way to restrain individuals. A full discussion of the use of drugs to restrain can be found in Chapter 3.

Proper medical practice limits the use of restraints to two purposes: first, to control behavior when a patient is out of contact with reality and a danger to himself or others, and second, to prevent patients from falling out of beds, chairs, etc., or from contaminating wounds or tearing off dressings. Even in this context, geriatricians such as Dr. Michael B. Miller, medical director, White Plains Center for Nursing Care, see the use of restraints as an admission of the failure of the nursing process.

Fire Chief Beman Biehl of Marietta, Ohio, testified that he and other rescuers had difficulty removing patients from a nursing home fire because they were tied to their beds. The fire, on January 9, 1970, claimed 32 lives.

An elderly Japanese woman was strapped to her wheel chair in a California nursing home "presumably for her own protection. She was unable to speak any English and no bilingual staff was present. She was ignored most of the time. One day she was found dead of suffocation because the straps were too tight."

Illinois Health Department files note one instance in which inspectors reported seeing a patient trying to go to the bathroom with a chair still tied to him with restraints. Other patients were also found tied to chairs.

One witness testified:

> A woman in a Minneapolis suburb remembers with vivid pain what happened when she took her mother, who had suffered a stroke, to a nursing home and returned the next morning to find her tied, without clothes, in bed in the midst of her own wastes. "I will never forget that sight," the woman wrote. "It's seared into my memory, seeing her struggling to free herself, crying out for someone to help her. She clung to me and cried like a child over and over again, 'Thank God you've come, thank God you've come.'

Reprisals Against Those Who Complain

The subcommittee received and verified reports of complaints by individual patients or nursing home personnel which resulted not in the correction of deficiencies but in reprisals against the complainants.

One letter which initiated a subcommittee probe of one Minneapolis home was a hastily typed plea to Senator Moss, stating:

> I hope you will come and visit me. Pretend you are a distant relative. I would talk on the phone but the walls have ears. I have to hurry because I am typing this letter in OT (occupational therapy) and I would hate to think what would happen if the home found out what I am doing.

Dr. David R. Holaday, chief of the Hospital and Medical Facility Branch of the Hawaii Health Department emphasized, "There is the fear of retribution from the homes. That's one reason families are reluctant to complain." Following are sworn statements from family members:

> • I complained to the head nurse about the other meals. Because I complained, the head nurse stopped helping my mother with the noon meals. So no one was feeding my mother. That's the way they handle things in nursing homes, if you complain about one thing, they just make it worse for you.

> • I was always afraid to say anything or complain about the home for fear of what might happen to my brother. I found myself lying about the home in front of their staff. I would tell them what a wonderful home they had and what wonderful care they gave their patients, though that was a lie, and I felt I had to lie for my brother's sake.

Lack of Eye Care, Dental Care, and Podiatry

Nursing home patients rarely can expect any sort of eye care. As a result, their already limited vision deteriorates. A study by the Lion's Sight and Service Foundation and the South Dakota Optometric Association found that appropriate care could have saved the sight of 67 percent of the legally blind nursing home patients in their study. The subcommittee also received many complaints that the eyeglasses of patients were inadequate, outdated, or lost. One nursing home employee testified:

> You can see over there [indicating], we have eyeglasses, and these are eyeglasses that are misplaced. Like they will take a patient's eyeglasses off at night and then when we come the

next day they are gone, and they get thrown in a box in a room, and because we don't remember what their eyeglasses look like and they aren't marked, we can't put them back on. Now and then we will gather the staff around and try to put glasses on patients.

Nursing home residents also need more attention to foot care. The aides and orderlies who are charged with doing this work told the subcommittee of having too much to do and not enough time to attend to the podiatry needs of patients.

> • There was another woman at the home that always walked around barefoot. She had palsy and I asked her why she walked around barefoot since it was so cold. She told me she couldn't put shoes on because they hurt her feet too much because no one would cut her toenails. Many people there seemed to have trouble with their toenails. Twice while I was there I saw this woman with the bad toenails fall and hurt herself badly. At least once she had to be taken to the hospital because of these falls.

> • Toenails and fingernails were never cut during my shift. They were supposed to be cut right after their bath, but the baths were not given on our shift. Many times the toenails got so long they grew into the toes underneath. The toenails of the majority of patients on the second floor were in that condition. I would say that approximately twenty-five patients had this condition.

A common assumption is that all nursing home residents have dentures and therefore, little need for dental services. Accordingly, few nursing home residents ever receive dental examinations. Studies and direct evidence received by the subcommittee, however, indicate that patients have substantial dental problems. The Harvard School of Dental Medicine, for example, reports that 77 percent of the patients in its study of nursing home residents had not seen a dentist since entry into a nursing home. A second study indicated that 54 out of 74 residents (78 percent) in one nursing home needed dental care, including extractions, restorations, and treatment of tumors. A third study of three nursing homes indicated that 64 percent of the 188 patients examined needed professional dental care.

Assaults on Human Dignity

Another common complaint is that in some facilities nursing home patients are treated like objects rather than people. A great many patients said they were given showers or baths in very hot or cold water as punishment. Others reported being left in the bath "for hours with the door open."

The following is a partial list of indignities suffered by some nursing home patients as taken from subcommittee files.

- Many of the seniors get embarrassed when we have to call maintenance men to help female patients into the bath. We put a gown over them when they get up, but they still get embarrassed. The other thing is that the maintenance men don't know how to handle the people well. They don't have any sensitivity towards the patients. They rush in and pull the patient out and scare them to death. This happens constantly. The personal modesty and privacy of the patient is not emphasized. Many rooms don't have screens. Even if there is a screen in the room, it isn't necessarily used.

- My mother was forced to stay in a room over my protests with a terminal cancer patient and the stench in the room was unbearable, partially due to the fact that the patient was not kept clean.

- One day when I was there an old man who was about 90 years old went into one of the ladies rooms by mistake. As a result of this mistake by this man, he was ridiculed and laughed at by many of the staff of the home. This same old man never had any underwear on. The home was hard up for underclothes, I guess. He had a big pair of trousers on that he wrapped around his waistline. He had trouble getting to the bathroom, and once he had a bowel movement accident while he was trying to get to the bathroom. This bowel movement rolled out of his pants and onto the floor. He tried to put it over into a corner with his shoe. Of course it got all over his shoe and everyone else was stepping in it. Nobody bothered to come and clean it up. Everybody would wait for somebody else to clean it up.

- There is also a pathetic shortage of clothes for the patients. It gets so bad that I have come on to work at 3 o'clock and their pants are held together, they are too small and the fly on their pants are held together by a chain of pins because they are so small.

• Also the linen in this home, they have the first floor, it is called the show floor...the laundry people in the laundry divide the linen. The better linen goes to the first floor, then the next in line goes to the second. Then all the rags and the raveled and stained linen goes to the third where the senile patients are.

Conclusion

It should be clear even from this cursory look that there are serious problems in the nursing home field. There is certainly some justification for the fears harbored by senior citizens. To what degree they are justified is the big question. Exactly how widespread are these abuses? Are the nursing homes described here the exception or the rule?

Chapter 3

Nursing Home Drugs: Pharmaceutical Russian Roulette

The topic of drug abuse consistently ranks as one of the most important domestic problems in the United States. In the public mind, it is almost always associated with young people. However, there is a hidden and scandalous problem of drug abuse among those who suffer the compound burden of illness and advanced age. It has been charged that as much as 40 to 50 percent of nursing home drugs may be administered in error. The tranquilizer has replaced Tender Loving Care in many of today's long term care facilities. Moreover, there is evidence of the use of nursing home patients as guinea pigs and abundant evidence of adverse reactions and death resulting from carelessly administered drugs.

The flow of drugs through America's 23,000 nursing homes is almost totally without controls. It is haphazard. It is inefficient. Most of all, it is dangerous to the patients who must trust others for their protection. The protection which should be coming from physicians, pharmacists, nurses, administrators, and government employees is nonexistent. In short, the use of drugs in a nursing home has become a kind of pharmaceutical Russian roulette.

THE NUMBERS

Senior citizens are ill three times as often as the younger population, are hospitalized three times as long, and spend three times as much for health care. Older Americans, in fact, constitute 10 percent of the population, but 30 percent of the nation's total health expenditures. These same ratios apply to pharmaceuticals. The aged account for 25 percent of all the prescriptions written in the United States. They spend about $103 a year for drugs, while most of us spend only $36.

Taking drugs has become a way of life for many elderly. Indeed, many owe their very lives to drugs. Modern miracle drugs, 70 percent of which were not available 20 years ago, have helped to set back mortality. But as more and more people live longer and longer, there is an ever-increasing number who suffer from multiple disabilities. These lingering maladies make large amounts of drugs necessary. The individuals who have the greatest number of medical disabilities and take the largest number of drugs are the aged in American nursing homes.

The best available statistics indicate that the average nursing home patient takes 4.2 different drugs and an average of 13 doses each day. More recent studies place the number of drugs taken at about 7 a day; some patients have been found taking 18 different drugs in one day and as many as 30 preparations in a nine-month period.

Drugs cost money. In the case of the average nursing home patient, it is over $400 a year. Most of this is paid on the patient's behalf by the government through either the Medicare or Medicaid program.

In short, the average nursing home patient will spend more than three times as much for drugs in a year as his senior citizen counterparts who are not institutionalized, and more than ten times as much as the average American. In all, the nation's over one million nursing home patients spent close to $500 million for drugs, or roughly five percent of the total nursing home expenditures in the United States.

The kinds and amounts of drugs flowing into nursing homes are truly alarming. Industry statistics and a GAO audit confirm that 37 percent of all pharmaceuticals sold to nursing homes were central nervous system drugs. The next largest category was anti-infective agents, with about 9 percent and then gastrointestinal drugs, with about 8 percent.

Clearly, the category of central nervous system drugs is the cause for alarm. This category contains tranquilizers, which constitute 19 percent of total drugs, and analgesics (painkillers), which make up 9 percent. The remaining 9 percent were sedatives and antidepressants.

It is startling, indeed, to learn that tranquilizers account for almost 20 percent of all drugs supplied to nursing homes, totaling about $100 million a year. But is is even more alarming to learn that fully one-half of all tranquilizers *and 10 percent of all drugs* used in homes were made up of the two most powerful tranquilizers—Thorazine and Mellaril. Each year, fifty million dollars worth of these two drugs flows into U.S. nursing homes despite the fact that the drugs are classified as antipsychotics, which means that they are to be prescribed only for individuals with serious mental illness. According to the AMA Drug

Evaluation Guide, these agents are poorly tolerated by nonpsychotic patients and the collateral risk of side effects is very great indeed.

DISTRIBUTION

Most Americans associate the initiation of medications with an examination by their physician, who directs a specific course of therapy and selects the drugs most useful for particular problems. But doctors are infrequent visitors to nursing homes; therefore, it is common practice in nursing homes today for nurses to call the patient's physician over the telephone. Drugs are then prescribed over the telephone.

Once authorized, how are the drugs distributed? Some few homes have their own pharmacists who oversee drug utilization. Another few utilize the unit dose distribution system. Unit dose means that each individual patient's medications are packaged by the pharmacist in a plastic bag containing the patient's name, the content and the strength of the drugs. The medications are sent to the home in a locked cart in which each patient has his own separate drawer. Only a 24-hour supply of medications is delivered to the home each day by the pharmacist.

Unfortunately, in most U.S. nursing homes, 30-day supplies of patient medications are stored in a drug closet (generally one per floor). Each patient may have from four to ten different prescription bottles which are opened daily to remove the required dose. These individual doses are placed in small cups identified with cards bearing the patient's name. Thereafter, a typical medication tray with the medications of perhaps 20 patients is taken to bedside. Each patient is then given the pills in the small paper cup identified by the namecard.

Thus, in a typical 100-bed nursing home, from 500 to 600 prescriptions would be required for patients at any one time. In a nine-month period, one home accumulated more than 850 different prescription bottles and over 17,000 doses of medication, not counting narcotics.

Understandably, this system has been described as inefficient and dangerous. The problem is amplified by the fact that, all too often, the management of drugs in nursing homes is left to untrained aides and orderlies. These individuals are hired literally off the street, in the words of one aide, "seldom knowing the difference between an aspirin and a mothball." The classic example was provided by Bill Recktenwald, chief investigator of Chicago's Better Government Association, who applied for a job as janitor and was hired as a nurse. Within minutes, he had the keys to the medication closet and the narcotics cabinet on his belt and was in charge of distributing medications to 37 patients in a Chicago nursing home.

Dan Henry, a Minneapolis nursing home orderly gave this similar testimony:

> My impression was that they would hire anyone off the streets who would come and could stand the conditions and would accept the wages they offered.
>
> I was given absolutely no training whatsoever in the passing of medication; however, I did this on a regular basis. Nurse's aides would also pass medications, and they did not have training in the effects of medications. All the nurses, nurse's aides, and orderlies had access to the narcotics cabinet. It was very common when there were drugs left over from a patient who had left or had died to re-use these drugs.

NURSING HOME STUDIES

Confronted with the widespread use of an inefficient and poorly controlled system of drug distribution, the infirm elderly are subject to a wide variety of drug abuses. The high degree of error in the existing distribution system has been revealed in studies by consumer groups, state and federal agencies, and schools of pharmacy and in testimony before the Subcommittee on Long Term Care.

Pharmacy School Studies

In late 1973, Dr. Allen M.K. Cheung, assistant professor of clinical pharmacy at the University of Southern California, documented a 22 percent rate of error in the distribution of drugs in a statistically valid sample of California nursing homes. Cheung says that even though the nurses knew that pharmacists would be looking over their shoulder, one out of every five doses was in error.

In a similar study, Professor Fred M. Eckel of the University of North Carolina School of Pharmacy documented a 69 percent rate of error, and later a 50 percent rate of error in the same study sample.

In these and other studies it is an error if a patient does not receive medications, or receives them at the wrong time or in improper combinations, or if undetected adverse reactions result.

The Nader Task Force Study

In one of the most detailed studies of nursing homes, the Nader Task Force on Nursing Homes, headed by Claire Townsend, reported:

Government statistics suggest widespread carelessness in the handling of drugs in nursing homes—drugs are administered incorrectly or not at all, drugs prescribed by physicians are allowed to continue too long, too many drugs are prescribed, or drugs are administered that have not been prescribed by a physician. Even more widespread is the practice of keeping patients under sedation to reduce the demands of the nursing staff.

General Accounting Office

Several studies by the GAO have confirmed these same facts. In an important 1966 audit relating to California nursing homes, GAO found that drugs were being given at the wrong time, in the wrong doses, sometimes to the wrong patient. In other cases, medications were not recorded, and sometimes patients did not receive the medication prescribed for them. In 1970, the GAO follow-up study found the same practices continuing and commented, "Actions taken by HEW and the states to correct the previously reported problems were generally ineffective."

The 1971 HEW Study

Further support for the premise that nursing home drugs are almost totally without controls comes from an extensive HEW study which reported:

- 37% of the patients taking cardiovascular drugs (digitalis or diuretics or both) had not had their blood pressure taken in over a year; for 25% of these there was no diagnosis of heart disease on the chart.
- 35% of the patients on phenothiazines had not had a blood pressure recorded in more than a year. Some were taking two and often three phenothiazine drugs concurrently. Some were on both psychotropic uppers and downers at the same time.
- A third of the patients being treated for diabetes mellitus had no diagnosis of diabetes on their charts. Over 10% of those receiving insulin or oral hypoglycemic agents were not on diabetic diets and a large number of these had not had a fasting blood/sugar test in more than a year.

Testimony before the Subcommittee on Long Term Care

If further evidence of the lack of controls on drugs were needed, it exists in volume after volume of the hearings conducted by the subcommittee. A few examples are illustrative. A nurse's aide offered this sworn statement:

> There is a constant problem with the giving out of medicines. There is an aide who has no nursing training who occasionally gives insulin injections. On one occasion she gave one diabetic patient an injection of insulin in the morning and did not mark it up in the day book. Later that morning an LPN gave her another injection, and I had to feed her sweets all day long.

Orderly Robert Shypulski testified:

> There is one incident that I would like to bring out, because I was called as a witness to it. There was an LPN named Mrs. B. who worked from 7 a.m. to 3:30 p.m. One day Mrs. D. noticed that there were three trays of medications that had been dumped in the waste basket. Mrs. B. had dumped them into a wastebasket. Mrs. D. called me as a witness. They put all the medication in a bag and called the head nurse. The next day Mrs. B. told the head nurse that she had not passed the medications because she did not feel that she should chase after all the patients. She didn't feel there was any sense in it.

In addition to statements from families, patients, and nursing home employees, testimony was also received from experts such as Dr. Allan Katz, president of the American Society of Consultant Pharmacists. Dr. Katz asserted that "the rate of errors for medications administered in long term care facilities is from 20 to 50 percent." He added that 60 percent of America's one million nursing home patients receive inadequate pharmaceutical services. After evaluating all the available evidence the subcommittee agreed with Dr. Katz's conclusion.

THE CHEMICAL STRAIGHT JACKET

Perhaps the most common and most devastating consequence of present inefficient drug distribution systems is the overuse of tranquilizers. Tranquilizers go by many names. Those most commonly used in nursing homes are called psychotropic drugs or antipsychotic agents; sometimes they go by their chemical name, phenothiazines or butyrophenones. Their proper use is to modify psychotic symptoms (mental illness) for purposes of decreasing aggressive or overactive behavior.

The report of the Nader Task Force on Nursing Homes charged that tranquilizers were given to patients mostly for staff convenience:

> In perhaps 50 percent of the letters we received there was mention of patients being put under sedation for no other reason than to simply keep them quiet and out of trouble.

This charge should not be surprising in view of claims made by manufacturers on behalf of such products. For example, Sandoz Pharmaceuticals, in their advertisements for the tranquilizer Mellaril, claims that the "far-reaching" effects of this drug will benefit the staff who will "find their work load greatly lightened as patient demands are replaced by a spirit of self-help and self-interest."

In 1970, Nelson Cruikshank, president of the National Council of Senior Citizens (NCSC), called upon Congress to investigate the "dangerous use of tranquilizer drugs on elderly nursing home patients simply to pacify them." He said:

> Excessive use of tranquilizers can quickly reduce an ambulatory patient to a zombie, confining the patient to a chair or bed, causing the patient's muscles to atrophy from inaction and causing general health to deteriorate quickly.
>
> Conscientious doctors may use tranquilizer drugs in a carefully administered program to help genuinely disturbed patients. However, it appears that many doctors, who are less than conscientious, give blanket instructions to nursing home staffs for the use of tranquilizer drugs on patients who do not need them.

In response, Senator Moss asked the U.S. General Accounting Office to conduct an audit of the kinds and amounts of drugs going to nursing home patients. The resulting GAO report confirmed industry data concerning the tremendous volume of tranquilizers flowing through nursing homes. As noted, they are far and away the largest category of nursing home medications, constituting almost 20 percent of the $500 million spent for drugs. Moreover, while the nursing home tranquilizer market is about $100 million a year, fully half of this amount went to purchase Thorazine and Mellaril, the two strongest available. While there are obviously many legitimate uses for tranquilizers, the sheer volume of these drugs going to nursing homes at least implies that they are given without controls.

William R. Hutton, executive director of NCSC, provided a great
deal of evidence that the overuse of these products is more fact than in-
ference. He offered these complaints from the thousands which NCSC
has received:

- Mr. T., Kansas City, Mo.—My mother is in a nursing home because
  she broke her hip and needs special care. I realize it's hard for her
  to get around but she acts like she's half dead. She tells me the
  medicine they give her makes her that way.
- Mrs. L., Los Angeles, Calif.—I would like to do something to help
  my mother who is 73. She has arthritis and has had to go to a nursing home. Ever since she went there, she acts like she's doped
  and I am afraid they keep her that way because then she doesn't
  need so much looking after.

Mr. Hutton's conclusion finds a great deal of support from the world-
famous British geriatrician, Dr. Lionel Z. Cousin. After studying
American nursing homes he said:

> There is a gross overuse of drugs in the care of the elderly
> in the United States. I think this is a failure on the part of in-
> ternal medicine to identify problems which result in dis-
> turbed behavior in the elderly patients. I suggest that with
> proper diet and environment that many disturbed patients
> can be calmed down. In fact, I think there is a good case for
> giving the tranquilizers to the staff and not the patients.

In order to accumulate more direct data on the question of indiscriminate tranquilization, Senator Moss made it the prime issue of
the Minneapolis hearings held in November 1971. Testifying at that
hearing, Daphne Krause produced more than 50 sworn affidavits from
nurses, patients, and families. It was this hearing which proved conclusively that in many nursing homes unlicensed aides and orderlies
had ready access to medications, including narcotics. In sworn
testimony, nursing home personnel admitted the common practice of
tranquilizing patients to keep them quiet. Nurse's aide Barbara Lace
testified:

> There is a heavy use of tranquilizers on our floor. We had a
> discussion about this once and I got kind of angry and told the
> nurse. There have been times when they woke the patients in
> order to give them tranquilizers so that the patients would

stay out of their hair. By keeping the patients drugged up, they are being turned into vegetables. Many of these patients are having psychological problems that are not being treated. They are medicated so that we don't have to deal with them.

Licensed Practical Nurse Kay Schallberg testified:

This nurse would also deliberately increase the dosage of a sedative much higher than the prescription in order to quiet down patients, but then she would put on the chart that she had administered the required dosage. She would take sedatives from the prescriptions of other patients in order to do this.

According to orderly Robert Shypulski:

Tranquilizers are used for everything. X was great for using tranquilizers. If you moved a muscle you got it. You could have dropped some of these people off the building and they wouldn't have blinked their eyes. It doesn't phase them anymore. We either posey (restrain) them or let them walk.

In presenting this information Daphne Krause told of her 6-year investigation of nursing homes in Minnesota, testifying that indiscriminate tranquilization was a common practice. She said:

For the beleaguered nurse's aide, tranquilizers are a happy solution. If the patients are sedated, they cause the staff few problems. The administrator is happy, too, because bedbound patients bring the highest rate of reimbursement.

Most nursing home administrators would dispute this claim. Dr. Charles Kramer is one who would not. As clinical director of the Plum Grove Nursing Home and assistant professor at the University of Illinois School of Medicine, he admitted, "Most tranquilizers in long term facilities are managed by nurses. I say that frankly and will probably get criticized for saying it." The word "nurse" is defined rather broadly in nursing homes to include unlicensed nurse's aides. There is no federal requirement to prohibit aides and orderlies from setting up and distributing drugs. Seeing an RN ordering a tranquilizer for an agitated patient, they may themselves feel qualified to do the same thing. The specter of aides prescribing tranquilizers on their own initiative is nothing short of hair-raising.

But the great tragedy in the use of tranquilizers is that it is the most active and aggressive patients who are the most likely to receive tranquilizers, and yet it is these patients who have the best chance for rehabilitation. Elaine Brody and Morton H. Kleban of the Philadelphia Geriatrics Center have written:

> In an institutional setting, there is a tendency on the part of the staff to expect conformity and cooperation. The "well adjusted" people are usually those who meet those standards. Aggressive, managerial individuals elicit negative reactions from others and therefore tend to be regarded as maladjusted, 'difficult,' and inflexible.
>
> Our data suggest very clearly that within this aggressive behavior is a force for self-improvement.

THE HIGH INCIDENCE OF DRUG REACTIONS

A few years ago, Dr. Margaret Mead sounded a warning in testimony before a Senate subcommittee: "We should be thinking about the tremendous health hazards of mixtures of drugs, of drugs that are administered in ignorance of the idiosyncrasies of the patient, of drugs that are administered in ignorance of the foods that are incompatible with them...." This admonition becomes more and more important as in recent years an increasing number of physicians, scientists, and pharmacists are turning their attention to the topic of adverse drug reactions. There is growing recognition of undesirable and toxic drug reactions that can occur, especially among the elderly, because of their reduced metabolic activity, altered central nervous system response, and reduced elimination of the drugs.

For these reasons, what should be a standard dose of medication for a middle-aged adult might well be an overdose for an older person. Moreover, scientists have documented variability in response to drugs taken by the elderly. Results are not always predictable in seniors. Similarly, the number and frequency of interactions and side effects for most drugs increase sharply with age. Edward S. Brady, associate dean of the School of Pharmacy, University of Southern California, wrote:

> The usual action of certain drugs may be influenced by chronic disease status of older people. Hence, usual dosages

might not be appropriate to this age group. For instance, in cases of impaired kidney function, the patient might not be able to excrete drugs from his system as rapidly as he should. Or, certain enzyme systems of the older person's body, affected by the slowdowns of aging, can greatly influence the results of drugs.

All of these problems are amplified when patients receive two or more drugs. The medical and pharmaceutical community is just beginning to learn that two drugs taken at the same time many nullify each other or produce harsh or unexpected results. In some cases, one drug will interact with (potentiate) another, so that the effect of the total is greater than the sum of the independent effects of either of the two substances taken individually. Obviously, the more drugs taken at the same time, the higher the chances of an adverse reaction. A patient taking five different drugs has a five percent chance of an adverse drug reaction. The odds increase to 45 percent when 20 drugs are taken.

Accordingly, nursing homes are the most likely place for adverse drug reactions. The average age of patients is 82 and they take from five to seven different drugs each day, some taken two and three times a day. Some patients take 20 or more drugs in the course of a month. Often, these drugs are taken for long periods of time. Finally, of the over 650,000 nursing home employees, comparatively few are licensed nurses (100,000). Unlicensed personnel (aides and orderlies) are for the most part untrained and unable to identify adverse reactions or side effects.

Following are some examples of common drug interactions:

- A most common interaction occurs between digitalis (a heart stimulant) and various kinds of diuretics (drugs increasing the output of urine). These drugs are commonly used in combination to treat congestive heart failure, a disease commonly present in the elderly. Many diuretics cause loss of potassium, increasing the toxic effect of digitalis on the heart. The usual result of this interaction would be heart rhythm irregularities which could result in death.
- Warfarin (a blood thinner) interacts with aspirin. Aspirin acts to potentiate the anticoagulant action of warfarin. The clinical result of this interaction would be hemorrhage due to enhanced warfarin action.

- Furazolidone (an antibiotic) can be nullified by Benzedrine (an amphetamine or "upper") or various foods containing tyramine, such as aged cheese, beer, or chicken livers.
- Aspirin can interact with alcohol leading to severe intestinal bleeding.
- Kanamycin and methicillin (two antibiotics) given simultaneously inactivate each other.
- Bisulfate, a preservative used to protect phenylephrine (an antihistamine and decongestant) will slowly inactivate penicillin (an antibiotic).
- Tranquilizers potentiate sedatives and analgesics (sleeping pills and pain killers).
- Antacids (i.e., Maalox) can sufficiently lower the rate of phenobarbital absorption.
- Laxatives speed passage of drugs through the gastrointestinal tract reducing the amount of the drug which is absorbed.

A detailed illustration of drug interaction is provided by Paul Lofholm, assistant clinical professor of pharmacy at the University of California, San Francisco:

> It is my experience, particularly in the nursing home area, that constipation is a problem not only because of the aging process, but also because the patient may be constantly bombarded by a number of constipating drugs. Here is a patient who fits a typical description: he is initially diagnosed as senile so is put on phenothiazine (tranquilizer) like Mellaril. A second drug, such as Elavil, is then added to his regimen perhaps because of depression. The patient has a little stomach problem, so Donnatal is added to take care of his stomach. In the meantime, drug-induced Parkinsonism occurs because of the administration of Thorazine or Stealazaine or Permatil, or Prolixin. This necessitates the use of an anti-Parkinson drug, such as Artance. Also, antacids which can be constipating are concurrently administered because of GI (gastrointestinal) problems; and finally iron salts or various minerals may be prescribed which are also binding. Now let's examine the patient's whole regimen. He is taking perhaps five or six or seven drugs which all have in common either a mineral effect or anticholinegic effect (an atropine-like side effect of constipation). Therefore, it is no wonder that the patient has difficulty, not because of his age, but also because of

the pharmacologic paralysis that occurs in the lower gut. Now, the central question is: does the patient need all of these drugs? Is there any way we can reduce the number of drugs to minimize particular side effects?[1]

The inherent dangers of drug interaction are all the more apparent after a quick look at the classes of the most commonly used drugs and their possible side effects. The following excerpts are taken from the American Medical Association Drug Evaluation Guide. As indicated, adverse reactions may be as mild as a headache or nausea, or as serious as convulsions and death.

Commonly Used Drugs

Diuretics (Diuril, Osmotrol, Lasix). These drugs are used to reduce the volume of extracellular fluid in order to eliminate edema (excessive accumulation of fluids) or prevent its developing. Adverse reaction may be either mild or dangerous, from headaches and nausea to dehydration and convulsions.

Sedatives (Seconal, Nembutal, Chloral Hydrates). When administered by day, and in small doses, sedatives may reduce emotional tension; in larger doses they induce sleep. Patients taking these drugs may show signs of lethargy. Prolonged use can lead to addiction, which the AMA drug guide notes "is more destructive to personality than narcotic dependence." Overdoses can result in death. Other drugs taken at the same time will increase the potency of sedatives. Among these are alcohol, antihistamines, and other central nervous system depressants.

Antianxiety Agents (Valium, Librium, Miltown). These drugs are used to suppress less severe manifestations of anxiety and tension. Adverse effects may include dizziness, impaired memory, and judgment. Some patients evidence paradoxical reactions; rather than becoming quiet, the disturbed patient becomes more violent. Addiction may result from the prolonged use of such agents and withdrawal symptoms may be severe (delirium and convulsions) when the drugs are terminated.

Antipsychotic Agents (Thorazine, Mellaril, Sparine). These drugs are useful in the treatment of acute and chronic psychosis. Ethical practice limits their use to relieving symptoms of mental illness or to alleviating delirium in individuals when antianxiety agents have failed.

The AMA Drug Evaluation Guide (1971 edition) practically overflows with caution in discussing the most powerful and most used tranquilizers, Thorazine, Mellaril, Sparine, and other so-called antipsychotics. It warns of severe side-effects, noting that it is important to recognize the side-effects of these drugs because "acute encephalitis, meningitis, tetanus and other neurological disorders have been diagnosed erroneously and patients have been treated accordingly."

Adverse reactions are not uncommon with these drugs, and great care must be used in the dosage levels employed. These drugs may produce Parkinsonian syndrome (tremors, shuffling gait, excessive salivation, mask-like faces); they may produce tardive dyskinesia, characterized by rhythmic movements of the tongue, jaw, and face, which persist even after the drug is discontinued. These drugs should be given to heart patients with great care because they may cause arrhythmias of the heart (erratic heartbeat), myocardial infarction (a type of heart attack), and death.

The AMA guide notes that the elderly are particularly susceptible to the detrimental side effects of antipsychotic agents. Good medical practice requires that their use be strictly time-limited and episodic, and that they be used as an adjunct to getting at the cause of the patient's agitation. In short, drugs have the potential for harm as well as for good. Their use needs to be carefully controlled and managed. The elderly, and particularly those in nursing homes, present special problems. Because of the large number of different drugs taken over protracted periods of time and the lack of personnel trained to deal with untoward effects, thousands of patients in long term institutions are prime candidates for adverse reactions.

The full impact of this problem has yet to be determined in nursing homes, but one ongoing study by Dr. James Coleman of Memphis, Tennessee provides insight. He wrote, "We nearly always find greater than 50 percent of the people in nursing homes are taking drugs which potentially interact and are subsequently quite dangerous." Despite strict hospital controls and the presence of trained personnel, 15 to 30 percent of the patients have one or more drug reactions during hospitalization. Drug misuse causes a total of 30,000 deaths annually, and the cost of drug-induced hospitalization is approximately $3 billion a year.

DRUG ADDICTION AMONG NURSING HOME PATIENTS

Most nursing home patients receive drugs over a protracted period of time, sometimes months and years. If a patient is taking narcotics, sedatives, antidepressants, or tranquilizers, there is a good possibility of addiction. Physical dependence on drugs is characterized by moderate to severe withdrawal symptoms. In some cases, delirium and convulsions result when the patient is taken off of the drug.

There are occasional references in the subcommittee's hearings to the problem of drug addiction among the elderly in nursing homes. The following is from the testimony of E.C. Morris, executive director of Planned Action for Community Elderly, Des Moines, Iowa.

> If I could have my files here and show you documented files — giving you as one example a man who was 94 years old, whose wife was 92. These two people were in our local hospital, under Medicare, they were there for 3 months. Their bills were over $12,000. The percentage of drugs in those cases was absolutely shocking. Now, I am a former administrator of Medicare in the Public Health Service. I know a little something about it. The lady passed away 3 days after I was appointed by the courts as their guardian conservator.
>
> We removed the gentleman; put him in a nursing home, and in 4 months' time this man's drug bill went from $20 to $104 a month for drugs.
>
> He went under the care of Dr. Harold Anderson, who does care about the elderly. We put him in another local nursing home — and for 3 weeks this man had to be held in restraint for drug removal. Today, I pay anywhere from $16 to $18 a month for his drugs.

There is no question that many of the drugs administered in nursing homes have at least the potential for addiction as well as other adverse side effects. One physician, who is also the executive director of a nursing home, has written:

> Many of these elderly people are dependent, if not truly addicted, on the medications that they are taking; this is easily verified by observing the patient when the doctor suggests discontinuing medications.
>
> ...We inform the elderly applicant prior to their arrival at the home that...we want to see how these old people fare without the ingestion of their multitudinous drugs....This is one of the few available opportunities we have for really 'drying' them out. I think that the popularity of our institution is really due in part to just that fact. Our clients really do seem to flourish.... I think that's why we are one of the few homes

for the aged which actually does graduate some of its residents back to society after they have been 'dried out' for several months, or perhaps a year.

While the suspicion lingers that addiction among nursing home patients is more frequent than anyone cares to imagine, there is little hard evidence. Without a doubt, this problem needs much more attention than it is receiving today. Perhaps part of the reason this situation has not been brought into sharper focus is the attitude of some professionals. The Nader task force reported, "One California physician, when told of an elderly lady's addiction to a painkiller Percodan replied: 'She is an old lady, let her enjoy it.'" Addiction in the elderly raises serious moral and ethical questions which should be faced head on and not swept under the rug of complacency.

HUMAN EXPERIMENTATION IN NURSING HOMES

In the normal course of developing new drugs, some experimentation with human beings is required. It is not uncommon for this testing to take place in nursing homes. Nursing homes provide many advantages to pharmaceutical companies:

1. The afflictions and infirmities which drugs are supposed to cure or treat abound in long term care facilities.
2. Patients tend to be long term, therefore, results can be carefully monitored.
3. The environment can be controlled to eliminate experimental variables.
4. Many nursing home patients have no family or friends, which reduces the possibility of law suits. And even if suits were to be brought, the measure of damages in U.S. Courts has traditionally been loss of earning power, life expectancy, and health—factors in which the elderly are peculiarly bankrupt.

It is obvious then, that while testing of drugs in nursing homes should not necessarily be discouraged, it should be permitted only under the strictest controls. The current absence of appropriate safeguards is a cause for great concern.

There are some 6,000 so-called "investigational" drugs being tested today. Americans like to think that testing involving human beings is carefully controlled, but the facts are to the contrary. Under the Food and Drug Administration's (FDA) rules, a company is free to begin tests in humans subject to FDA veto, 30 days after notifying the agency of its intention. In practice, the FDA permits clinical testing in humans to begin after only two weeks of animal studies—*even before those animal studies have been evaluated.*

These facts and others came to light in a September 1973 report by the GAO charging that the FDA had failed to protect patients in whom medications were being tested for safety and effectiveness. Senator Abraham Ribicoff, who released the report, charged that pharmaceutical companies had failed to establish safe testing procedures and had resisted FDA regulation.

The GAO provided startling examples of pharmaceutical companies' failure to notify the FDA after learning that people were exposed to drugs which caused adverse reactions in animals. Time lags in giving the FDA crucial data ranged from one month to a year and a half. In one case, Ayerest Laboratories waited 19 months before reporting to the FDA the conclusions of a British study showing a possible connection between cancer in mice and its experimental drug, Pronetholol. In another case, the GAO charged that the company had refused to inform the doctors conducting the tests in humans of tests showing cancerous tumors in animals. Ayerest also disregarded three FDA orders to halt testing of its experimental drug, Practolol. In yet another case, E.R. Squibb and Sons halted tests on 324 patients receiving Cinanserin (once described by a Squibb executive as a drug looking for a condition to treat) after liver tumors developed in long term tests with rats, but Squibb refused to undertake patient follow-up.

The GAO study has relevance in the nursing home context as well. The subcommittee received several complaints charging improper controls. Most of these involved the question of "informed consent." Was the patient capable of understanding the situation and knowingly give permission?

One such case involved the drug "Anavar" (developed by G.D. Searle and Co.) in which the patient's informed consent was established by an "X" on the consent statement. Ralph Nader and his Task Force on Nursing Homes investigated the case in some detail. Testifying before the subcommittee in December of 1970, they said:

> Drug companies frequently carry out experimental drug research on nursing home patients. One woman's report of an experiment involving her mother is a striking example of the opportunities for abuse that can occur. The case is unusual only in that the family of the patient made exhaustive inquiries

following her death and found that no one—the government, the attending physician, or the home—was adequately protecting the patient.

Unknown to the family (the daughter had expressly told the attending physician not to allow her mother to be given experimental drugs), the nursing home and attending physician approved the patient, among others, for the experiment. The patient's "consent" was gained; she marked an X on a consent statement.

After taking the drug for about 6 months, the patient became critically ill. Medical diagnosis never confirmed the cause of the illness; no move was made to find out whether the experimental drug had caused or contributed to the illness; the drug continued to be given.

Two months later, the woman died. Both the home and the coroner who filled out the death certificate refused to tell the family exactly how or why the woman died. The home has refused to release the woman's medical records to her family.

The family did obtain a record of the drugs given the patient and discovered that she was taking an experimental drug. When they demanded to know why they had not been consulted, the home produced a "consent" document marked with the patient's X. The patient had been judged senile by her doctor who recommended that she live in an institution. Nonetheless, the home maintained and the FDA concurred, that the "consent" of a person medically diagnosed as senile was sufficient.

The family further discovered that the woman's doctor believed the drug given was already approved and not as an experimental drug. He, therefore, made no attempt to see whether the drug was having ill effects on the patient. In this case, according to the daughter, certain allergies and an edema condition made it possible that the drug could have been highly dangerous for her mother.

The Anavar example points out clearly the need for the FDA to exercise particular vigilance in the case of drug experimentation with nursing home patients. The FDA should require a strict standard of consent where the infirm elderly are involved, and pharmaceutical companies should be held accountable for the well-being of these patients.

Conclusion

It is clear that an incredible volume of drugs flows through America's long term care facilities by way of an antiquated distribution system. The system provides easy access to medications by all nursing home employees and looks to untrained and unlicensed personnel to set up and distribute medications. The result is that 20 to 40 percent of the drugs given to nursing home patients are administered in error. Moreover, there is a high incidence of adverse reactions, including addiction. Indiscriminate tranquilization to make patients easier to handle appears to be common. Finally, nursing home patients are sometimes used as human guinea pigs, raising serious questions about whether they gave "informed consent" for such procedures.

All in all, the lack of controls on nursing home drugs is one of the most serious problems that confronts nursing homes. It is a desperate situation which cries out for reform. It will require concerted effort from physicians, nurses, administrators, and pharmacists to take the gamble out of taking drugs in a nursing home.

Chapter 4

Nursing Home Fires: A Chronic Condition

With the coming of winter and the stoking of furnaces to remove the chill of the north wind, one phenomenon is just about as predictable as snowfall, and that is the continuing chronicle of nursing home fires. There were some 9,000 nursing home fires in 1976, an average of 25 a day for each day of the year. Most of the fires resulted only in property damage, some six million dollars' worth. An estimated 500 patients died in single-fatality fires, which seldom make the news and which often are not even reported. There were four major tragedies known as multiple-death fires, in which a total of 41 patients died.

As shocking as it seems, this sorry record is nothing new. Between 1957 and 1966, 287 patients died in multiple death nursing home fires. In the past ten years, 232 people died in nursing home fires. As early as 1964, representatives of the National Fire Protection Association (NFPA) testified before the subcommittee, "When one compares this fatal fire record with the record of fatal fires in other property, it becomes clear that nursing homes are extremely unsafe places to live." The spokesmen pointed out that six patients died in nursing home fires for every one in a hospital fire. Actually, this ratio is much higher for the last ten years because there have been only about 20 deaths in multiple death hospital fires over the past ten years as contrasted with the 232 who died in nursing homes.

The serious problem of nursing home fires has also been recognized by the President's Commission on Fire Safety and Control which singles out nursing home patients as cause for "special and growing concern." "It is a blemish on the American conscience that those who contributed to our prosperity are allowed to live their retirement years where even minimal fire safeguards are absent." The Subcommittee on Long Term Care agreed, charging in its August 1975 report that "despite much progress in recent years, nursing homes and related facilities still rank number one in the list of unsafe places to be from a fire safety point of view." Table 4-1 provides graphic evidence in support of this conclusion.

Table 4-1 Multiple-Death Fires* in Nursing Homes and Related Facilities as Reported to the National Fire Protection Association (1951-1976)

Date and Location	Number Killed
January 30, 1951: Hogwam, Wash.	21
June 18, 1951: Colesville, Md.	4
May 1, 1952: Bradford, Conn.	3
October 31, 1952: Hillsboro, Mo.	20
January 14, 1953: Warren, Pa.	7
January 25, 1953: Billings, Mont.	6
March 29, 1953: Largo, Fla.	33
February 19, 1954: Watervliet, Mich.	8
May 7, 1954: Houston, Tex.	3
September 17, 1954: Kincaid, Kan.	7
December 6, 1954: Germantown, Md.	7
December 19, 1954: New Orleans, La.	6
February 11, 1955: Brownwood, Tex.	4
March 5, 1955: Edmeston, N.Y.	3
December 17, 1955: Beaumont, Tex.	4
June 22, 1956: Princeton, N.J.	3
July 30, 1956: Puxico, Mo.	12
February 13, 1957: Council Bluffs, Iowa	15
February 17, 1957: Warrenton, Mo.	72
June 23, 1957: Chicago, Ill.	3
December 12, 1957: Bardstown, Ky.	5
January 6, 1959: Martinsburg, W. Va.	5
January 30, 1959: Glen Ellyn, Ill.	9
March 13, 1959: Aurora, Ill.	4
February 1, 1961: Washington, D.C.	7
December 16, 1961: Sheridan, Wyo.	4
December 31, 1961: Roundup, Mont.	3
April 2, 1962: Yeadon, Pa.	9
August 24, 1962: Electra, Tex.	5

*A multiple-death fire is defined as one in which 3 or more people receive injuries which cause death within one year of the fire.

Table 4-1 (Continued)

Date and Location	Number Killed
December 20, 1962: Hudson, Mass.	9
February 1, 1963: Mount Vernon, Mo.	3
September 17, 1963: Pinehurst, Ida.	7
November 23, 1963: Fitchville, Ohio	63
January 2, 1964: Columbia, Miss.	3
March 12, 1964: Cleveland, Ga.	4
July 23, 1964: Ardmore, Okla.	4
October 23, 1964: Syracuse, N.Y.	4
October 30, 1964: Colusa, Cal.	7
December 17, 1964: Winfield, Ill.	4
December 18, 1964: Fountaintown, Ind.	20
January 16, 1965: Near Linn, Mo.	5
March 27, 1965: South Boston, Mass.	3
February 7, 1966: Bay Shore, L.I., N.Y.	6
February 8, 1966: Clinton Corner, N.Y.	4
February 8, 1967: North Strafford, N.H.	4
May 20, 1967: Princeton, W. Va.	4
September 23, 1967: Tucson, Ariz.	4
January 18, 1969: Greenville, Miss.	7
March 18, 1969: Marshalltown, Iowa	5
April 11, 1969: Fisherville, Va.	3
July 3, 1969: Harding, Pa.	4
January 9, 1970: Marietta, Ohio	31
January 14, 1971: Buechel, Ky.	10
September 15, 1971: Salt Lake City, Utah	6
October 19, 1971: Honesdale, Pa.	15
January 26, 1972: Lincoln Heights, Ohio	10
April 4, 1972: Rosecrans, Wis.	10
May 5, 1972: Springfield, Ill.	10
November 27, 1972: Kearney, Neb.	4
January 8, 1973: Madison, Wis.	3
January 14, 1973: Charleston, W. Va.	6
January 15, 1973: Addison, N.Y.	3
January 29, 1973: Pleasantville, N.J.	10
April 21, 1973: New Haven, Ky.	3
September 12, 1973: Philadelphia, Pa.	11
December 4, 1973: Wayne, Pa.	15
August 16, 1974: Brookhaven, Miss.	6

Date and Location	Number Killed
September 9, 1974: St. Joseph, Mo.	7
January 30, 1976: Chicago, Ill.	23
February 4, 1976: Cicero, Ill.	8
June 17, 1976: Roanoke, Va.	4
November 27, 1976: Philadelphia, Pa.	6
February 17, 1977: Zion, Ill.	3

WHY ARE NURSING HOMES A SPECIAL FIRE SAFETY PROBLEM?

The obvious answer to the question lies in the characteristics of nursing home patients. They are very old; the average age is 82. They suffer from four or more major disabilities. The great majority of them are mentally impaired. Less than half can walk without assistance; most would have difficulty climbing stairs or performing more complex movements, such as climbing out a window in case of fire.

Age often brings with it impairment of one or more of the senses essential to detection of fire and to taking action to escape. Sensory impairments can lead to disorientation, which can be particularly deadly in a fire. The senses most commonly affected are hearing, vision, and smell.

To add to these problems, the elderly do not withstand the effects of heat well. They are more susceptible to burns and to respiratory damage through inhalation, and they do not tolerate smoke and gases as well as younger people. In low concentrations, gases irritate, causing gasping (and the inhalation of more gases) and blinding. In higher concentrations, they are fatal poisons. The most common cause of death in fires is carbon monoxide, an odorless, colorless gas which is a product of incomplete combustion. A concentration of 1.28 percent can cause death in three minutes.

Finally, the elderly are more susceptible to shock. Shock is unpredictable and often inexplicable physiological reaction to disaster or emergency. It may be brought on by the sight of a fire or the fear of it. In the elderly, it can bring about heart failure.

In testimony before the Subcommittee on Long Term Care, Richard Steven, managing engineer of the National Fire Protection Association, summarized his experience, calling nursing home patients themselves the greatest obstacle to safety:

> Fire experience has shown that the primary problem in providing a reasonable degree of life safety from fire in this type of occupancy is the patient himself.
>
> The facts show that the patient is generally incapable of any act of self-preservation in an emergency situation due either to his own mental or physical infirmities or to conditions which are forced upon him. He will frequently observe the starting and progression of a fire without taking any action of self preservation or of sounding an alarm to alert others. The patient often will not follow verbal instructions to evacuate the building and, if forced to leave, will often struggle with those who attempt to move in. Furthermore, once evacuated, a patient is very apt to reenter the building if not restrained. This means that evacuation of these places — the usual course to follow in a fire emergency in a building — becomes practically an impossibility with the limited staff available.
>
> Since many of the patients do not possess the mental and physical abilities that they once enjoyed, they are apt to be the originators of fires either through acts of carelessness, overt acts, or physical inability to deal with a situation.
>
> It is my opinion, therefore, that the patient is the primary reason that these places are unique amongst all occupancies when considering the problem of life safety from fire.

As Mr. Stevens implies, dangers from nursing home fires are not caused solely by the inherent mental and physical characteristics of the patients themselves. About 33 percent of nursing home fires were caused by smoking or matches; heating or electrical problems followed next with 18 and 15 percent respectively. Eight percent were labeled "suspicious" — a suggestion that arson was the suspected or assigned cause. Most fires began in patients' rooms (35 percent) and most took place from midnight to 6 a.m. (42 percent). Some 35 percent of nursing home fires occurred in wood frame buildings, while only 3 percent happened in fire-resistant buildings.

Restraints and Sedatives

The use of restraints or sedatives must be carefully monitored. In fires, both present special problems to the patients and to the firefighters trying to evacuate them. Sedation played a major role in the Honesdale, Pennsylvania fire (October 19, 1971), in which 15 died. NFPA records show that the nurse could not wake patients to warn them because she had given them all tranquilizers or sedatives just an hour before the outbreak of the fire. In a similar case, a nurse's aide on duty at the time of the Marietta, Ohio fire (January 9, 1970), in which 31 people died, reported: "I think they must have gotten it in their sleep because I heard the morgue say that they never got a more relaxed bunch of corpses." Restraints contributed to the loss of life in the same two fires. Fire Chief Beman Biehl, of Marietta, Ohio, testified to having to use his pocket knife to cut through restraining straps which impeded rescue efforts.

Inadequately Trained Personnel

Another significant cause of nursing home fires is the inability of nursing home personnel to cope with the fire emergency. Representatives of the nursing home industry have often noted the high turnover rate (75 percent for nurse's aides) as an excuse for the inability of nursing home personnel to respond to emergencies. In some cases personnel are simply untrained; there are no fire drills or fire evacuation plans. A particular problem is the shortage of supervision at night. Mr. Stevens notes: "Even in situations where employee training is outstanding, human frailties are generally inevitable during emergencies."

The performance of nursing home employees has been a central issue in each and every fire investigated by or reported to the subcommittee. In the Lincoln Heights, Ohio fire (January 26, 1972), only one nurse's aide was on duty when the fire broke out at 2:30 a.m. In the Rosecrans, Wisconsin fire (April 4, 1972), there was no one on duty when the fire began at 11:15 p.m. In Springfield, Illinois (May 5, 1972), only two employees were on duty at 5:35 a.m. when the fire started.

The Marietta fire also highlighted human error. In rescuing the patient in whose room the fire started, aides failed to close the door of the fire room behind them. Experts stated that if the door had remained shut, there would have been no deaths in that fire. An open door also contributed to the loss of life in the Salt Lake City fire

(September 15, 1971). Professor Irving Einhorn, of the University of Utah's Flammability Research Center, testified that if the crucial door at the top of the stairway had been closed, survival time on the upper floor would have been increased from three minutes to about ten minutes.

Housekeeping and Maintenance

Several nursing home fires have been attributed to improper maintenance and housekeeping. Maintenance is used here in the sense of keeping machinery and electrical equipment in good working order. The Honesdale fire, for example, was initially blamed on a defective clothes dryer. Two fires—Fountaintown, Indiana and Lincoln Heights, Ohio—were the result of defective heating systems. The cause of the Fitchville, Ohio (claiming 63 lives), and the Warrenton, Missouri fires (claiming 57 lives) was defective electrical wiring.

It is especially important to remove flammable material from storage closets that are easily accessible to patients. Wastepaper baskets and laundry chutes become less hazardous if emptied often. Trash and debris, if allowed to accumulate, are a natural fire hazard. The Marietta fire began in a plastic wastebasket full of refuse. The Kearney, Nebraska fire started in a pile of clothes ignited by a cigarette; the Wayne, Pennsylvania fire in a clothes closet; and the Brookhaven, Mississippi fire in a supply closet. A patient with access to a flammable liquid started the fire in Salt Lake City, Utah which claimed six lives.

Smoking

Smoking and matches stand out as the principal cause of nursing home fires. Some 33 percent of all fires are caused by smoking. Smoking has been the primary reason for the nursing home fires in Rosecrans and Madison, Wisconsin; Kearney, Nebraska; and Marietta, Ohio.

In Marietta, experts concluded that either the patient was trying to smoke unassisted, or an aide had emptied a "hot" cigarette into a plastic wastebasket filled with paper. Because of the Marietta experience and the general inability of the comparatively few nurses and aides to supervise patients' smoking, some experts are in favor of banning patients' smoking, and some are in favor of banning smoking in patients' rooms. Mayor John Burnworth of Marietta testified:

> However, now let me get to the root of the problem. I submit to you that, had smoking not been permitted in this nursing home, this fire would not have occurred. I strongly urge that laws be enacted which would prohibit any type of smoking in nursing homes, hospitals, or for that matter, any place that houses persons who are totally or partially immobile except in areas specially designed and set aside for the purpose of smoking.
>
> It is my opinion that no employee, patient or visitor should ever be allowed to smoke in a patient's room, under any circumstances.

State Fire Marshal Samuel Sides concurred in this recommendation and recommended its enactment to the Ohio legislature.

PRECAUTIONS AGAINST FIRE

The series of Senate hearings on nursing home problems in 1965 revealed that patients were essentially without protection against fire except in a few progressive states. The result was the introduction of a bill requiring nursing homes participating in the Medicaid program to comply with a set of minimum federal standards.

The proposal, which was enacted in December 1967, requires nursing homes to be in compliance with the Life Safety Code of the National Fire Protection Association. The code is a comprehensive series of requirements developed after years of experience by the nation's leading fire safety experts. The code stresses saving lives, not simply minimizing structural damage. Compliance with the 1973 edition of the code is now required by law.

The code incorporates all elements of fire safety technology. Among these components are protection, detection, extinguishment, confinement, and control. Confinement and control both relate to building structure. It is a simple fact that a nursing home built of brick will burn less readily than one made of wood. One technique relied upon is "compartmentation," constructing a building into completely enclosed segments; thus a fire in one area of a facility cannot spread to another section.

Protection involves developing procedures and plans to insure evacuation. Detection is extremely important. The length of time between a fire's beginning and its discovery is a crucial factor in saving lives and limiting damage. There are three types of detectors in use at the present time. The first is activated by heat, the others by smoke and gas. Such detectors play an extremely important role, particularly when they are connected directly to a local fire department. But they are not the total answer. The Salt Lake City nursing home fire in 1971 provided a classic lesson. The detection system was connected directly to the fire department; it could not have functioned more effectively, but still, six patients died. Fire Marshall Ben Andrus explained:

> Our district chief in this area was coming back from another alarm at approximately eight-tenths of a mile away from the Lil-Haven when the warning on the dispatch came in. This dispatch took 50 seconds from the time they made the preliminary warning until they completed and gave the time as 0041 or 12:41 a.m. The district chief arrived at 0042, or 58 seconds from the conclusion of the preliminary warning. The first engine company arrived at 0043, 1 minute behind him, and the first ladder company arrived at 0044. So within 3 minutes of dispatch we had a chief officer, one pumper and one ladder company, with a special dispatch on the second ladder company. The fire took approximately 10 minutes to get under control.

Senator Moss commented that the fire department could not have reacted more quickly if they had set the fire themselves. With Utah's governor, Calvin Hampton, he called for the enactment of legislation requiring all nursing homes to install automatic sprinkler systems. In Utah, the governor's executive order took effect immediately. Some five years and several fires later, Congress had not acted on Senator Moss's proposal, a bill later introduced in the House by Claude Pepper, chairman of the House Aging Committee. The proposal for nursing home sprinkler systems has received universal endorsement from the National Safety Council, the National Fire Protection Association, the Fire Marshals of North America, the Joint Committee on the Accreditation of Hospitals, the American Health Care Association, and the Special Studies Subcommittee of the Government Operations Committee of the House of Representatives.

Some nursing home administrators have also endorsed sprinkler systems, thinking that they constitute the ultimate protection, making detection, compartmentation, and the like unnecessary. The NFPA rejects this notion, claiming that the systems should be used in combination with other precautions. Dr. Einhorn adds that while sprinklers are no panacea (he is a strong advocate of smoke detectors as well), they are by and large the difference between life and death to nursing home patients. The Life Safety Code requires sprinklers in all types of facilities except fire resistant, single-story, protected, noncombustible buildings. In its June 1976 audit, the U.S. General Accounting Office joined Congressman Pepper and Senator Moss in recommending that even these homes be required to install sprinklers.

NEW CONCERNS

There is another area which the subcommittee felt was not adequately covered in the Life Safety Code—the lack of adequate flammability, smoke generation, and toxicology standards for carpets and furnishings. The issue of the flammability of carpeting first came to the subcommittee's attention when it emerged as the central cause for the 1970 Marietta, Ohio nursing home fire deaths. The carpet backing was a rubber foam substance that produced large amounts of thick black smoke which caused most of the 31 Marietta deaths. At the Senate hearings on this fire, HEW and the Department of Commerce both promised to issue forthright standards concerning carpet flammability. (HEW standards would, of course, relate to nursing homes, and the Commerce Department standards would apply to carpet made available to the general public.)

HEW already had one standard on its books which was acceptable to experts—the E-84 Tunnel Test. It is an attempt to measure how fast an item burns compared to asbestos, which is assigned a score of zero, and red oak, which scores 100. Under Hill-Burton standards, carpeting must score 75 or less on the Tunnel test. The carpet industry has fought the promulgation of this standard by HEW for at least the past six years, arguing instead for a weaker standard called "the pill test." In the pill test, a small methenamine tablet is placed on a carpet specimen and ignited. This tablet burns with a small (approximately match size) flame for about 100 seconds. If the specimen burns three inchs in any direction, it has failed the test.

In October of 1972, Senator Warren G. Magnuson, chairman of the Senate Commerce Committee took the Senate floor to denounce HEW and the Department of Commerce for refusing to go along with a stricter test for flammability. He charged that the Nixon Administration promised to postpone effective regulations for carpeting in order to obtain a campaign contribution of $94,580 from the carpet industry. He told the Senate that President Nixon's former campaign finance chief, former Secretary of Commerce Maurice Stans, "set up a hush-hush high level White House meeting to assure that such effective regulation would not be forthcoming." William N. Letson, general counsel of the Department of Commerce, acknowledged the meeting but denied that it was a secret or that any favors were offered. Whatever the reason, the Department of Commerce is substantially in breach of its obligations to Congress and the general public under the Flammable Fabrics Act at least with respect to carpet standards.

During the June 3, 1976 joint hearings of the House and Senate Aging Committees, HEW officials proposed the "pill tests" as the standard for patients' rooms. Clearly, this standard is anemic and provides patients with little protection. The great majority of the carpeting produced in this country (including that which caused the deaths of 31 patients in the Marietta nursing home) will pass the pill test.

The dispute over carpeting standards also brings into focus the lack of emphasis on smoke generation and toxicology in HEW standards. Tests show that burning synthetic fibers such as acrylic and nylon carpeting produce lethal gases which can kill within minutes, even at room temperature; mortality increases with higher temperatures and greater exposure time. Some 50 percent of all nursing home deaths and about 5,000 of the total 8,000 fire deaths nationally are attributed to smoke inhalation.

Actually, comparatively little is known about what products make smoke lethal. Dr. Ann W. Phillips, of Harvard University and Massachusetts General Hospital, testified that only three people survived the Boston Coconut Grove fire and they were people who covered their faces with a little cloth. Since smoke can penetrate most fabric, it is not known what particles or gas might have been repelled by the screening. It is generally agreed that the thick black smoke was also the killer in Marietta, but it is not known what products the smoke might have been carrying. It is enough to state that smoke replaced the oxygen needed for life. Carbon monoxide, credited with most fire deaths, usurps the rightful place of oxygen on hemoglobin molecules in the blood and further reduces the amount of oxygen carried to the victim's brain, distorting judgment and impairing coordination so that escape is impossible. But there is more to it than that.

Carbon dioxide is also released in a fire. Although nontoxic, it stimulates respiration, which increases the intake of other toxic gases. Sulfur dioxide, a heavy, pungent gas extremely toxic to humans, is also released by burning synthetics. Combined with water, it forms extremely corrosive sulfurous acid. Hydrocarbons are also commonly produced. Hydrogen chloride, vinyl chloride, and phosgene are often present. Phosgene is a deadly gas used in warfare. Hydrogen chloride combined with water produces hydrochloric acid. Another gas released is hydrogen fluoride, which is lethal in and of itself, but when added to water, it will burn flesh like hydrofluoric acid. Hydrogen cyanide is yet another gas that is produced.

It is alarming that so little is known about the toxic consequences of combustion. The irony is that in the efforts to reduce flammability, the result may be to increase the amount of smoke, which Dr. Einhorn contends is 100 times more dangerous. In a nursing home this means that plastic, vinyl, foam rubber padding, furniture, carpet backing, or even some sprays marketed to make fibers flameproof may increase the production of smoke and the chance of death due to smoke inhalation. One of the many lessons from Marietta is that products made from petroleum not only burn like petroleum, but release deadly gases.

Unfortunately, the National Bureau of Standards and the Department of Commerce have placed their major emphasis on flammability and made little attempt to analyze the gases produced in a fire. The folly of this policy for all Americans, young and old alike, can be seen from the events subsequent to the December 8, 1972 crash of a United Airlines 727 aircraft at Midway Airport in Chicago. Dr. Andrew J. Tolman, a medical examiner, disclosed that sufficient quantities of cyanide were found in the blood stream of some victims to have caused death. Dr. Tolman said that the victims inhaled the cyanide fumes along with the smoke from the fire caused by the crash. He attributed the poisonous fumes to burning foam rubber in the seats and to plastic coating used on the curtains and seats.

In short, there is a need to consider the toxicological as well as the flammability properties of materials and furnishings used in nursing homes. Prevention requires an attack on many fronts—construction, furnishing, maintenance, training of personnel, and early detection.

The Lack of Enforcement

Perhaps even more troubling than these shortcomings in existing regulations is the lack of enforcement of laws and regulations that have been on the books since December of 1967. The provisions of the Life Safety Code have never really been enforced, which may help explain why the death toll in multiple-death nursing home fires has not dropped substantially in the past ten years.

The extent of this nonenforcement is staggering. In May of 1971, the GAO released a report charging that 50 percent of the nursing homes evaluated in its three-state sample had serious fire safety deficiencies.

Four years later, the GAO revealed that 72 percent of the nursing homes in its 11-state sample had one or more violations of major Life Safety Code provisions.

There is little argument about the validity of the GAO's findings. HEW's own statistics show a similar pattern. In 1974, HEW reported that 59 percent of all "skilled nursing facilities" had serious deficiencies. A year later, after an exhaustive study, HEW reported that two-thirds of these homes had "several (four or more) deficiencies," and in 1976, 47 percent.

According to the GAO, not only are standards not being enforced, there is a lack of uniformity of interpretation and application of the Life Safety Code by state surveyors who inspect nursing homes applying federal standards. The GAO pointed out that only 22 percent of those doing fire inspections had backgrounds qualifying them to do so; 78 percent were nurses, sanitarians, and members of other professions, including state police or detectives.

HEW's usual excuse for not enforcing standards is that Medicaid is a state-administered program and that they can do little to discipline a state which is lax in enforcement of the law. HEW claims (erroneously) that the only weapon it has is to withhold funds from an entire state, meaning that they have no authority to withhold federal funds to specific nursing homes. The states usually respond that they would like to enforce standards, but that would mean closing homes—a long and tedious process. They add that they are reluctant to close a home because they have "no place else to put the patients."

In the authors' view, these attitudes were merely excuses. In temporizing with the law to please the present generation of nursing home operators or those states loathe to close homes and relocate patients, HEW has been guaranteeing that the U.S. will be plagued by the continuing chronicle of nursing home fires.

Chapter 5

Profiteering: Services to the Needy by the Greedy

Just how profitable is the nursing home industry? To what extent are nursing home operators profiteers? To what extent do they seek unreasonable profits at the expense of their patients?

Nursing home owners and administrators have continually charged that public assistance rates are inadequate. As evidence, they point to the rates they charge their private patients, which, they say, reflect what adequate reimbursement should be. They continually contend that private paying patients are subsidizing the indigent patients. They defend the practice of adding ancillary charges onto the basic rates charged private paying patients. They have even argued that kickbacks from pharmacists and other suppliers, if they exist at all, are caused by low Medicaid rates. This same rationale leads most administrators to "understand" how a few operators could resort to asking for under-the-table payments to supplement public assistance rates—a violation of the law. All of this they charge while steadfastly refusing to allow consumer groups, state government, and/or senate investigative teams access to the financial records which could conclusively prove their case.

Critics of the industry charge that Medicaid rates are adequate and even present the possibility of generous profits. They charge that administrators are profiteers who see private paying patients as a golden windfall. Many charge that the profit motive is inconsistent with good care and the values of the American society. Finally, they have little patience with the failure of nursing home administrators to allow access to their financial statements. They argue that since more than half of nursing home revenues comes from public coffers, the public has a right to see how its money is spent. They add that if such financial data shows losses, they will support increases in rates for the industry.

While the issue is complex and extremely sensitive, the studies which have been undertaken and the weight of informed opinion generally give credence to the charge that the nursing home industry is immensely profitable.[1]

THE IMMENSE PROFITABILITY OF THE NURSING HOME INDUSTRY

From 1960 through 1976, expenditures for nursing home care have increased 2,000 percent from $500 million to $10.5 billion. Study after study indicates that this meteoric pattern of growth will continue and that nursing homes will continue to be highly profitable.

Advice to Bankers

In 1964, George Wells of the Federal Reserve Bank of Boston submitted a thesis at the Stonier Graduate School of Banking conducted by the American Banker's Association. The thesis became widely circulated under the title "Financing Nursing Homes." Mr. Wells wrote in his introduction that the purpose of his work was to consider whether the financing of nursing homes is a sound investment for commercial banks. Mr. Wells advised his fellow bankers to invest. His detailed study went so far as to warn bankers not to lend unless the owner was taking an active role in management, and advised that a 75- to 100-bed home was the most economical. In terms of profits he wrote, "Based on interviews with bankers, government officials and others listed in the bibliography (nursing home spokesmen included), a 20 percent throwoff for debt service and profit is common. A net profit (after income tax) of from 10 to 20 percent of gross income is not uncommon." He concluded, "An efficiently operated nursing home is a sound investment for time deposits." This report was presented to the subcommittee during its 1965 hearings. It was a major factor in our decision to document the truth about nursing home profitability in its 1969-1976 hearings.

The Chicago Hearings

The April 2 and 3, 1971 hearings held by the subcommittee in Chicago, Illinois focused on several questions, including the profitability of certain nursing homes which repeatedly violated state and city standards. The data was difficult to obtain. Operators would not come forth voluntarily. Finally, congressional subpoenae were issued. Benjamin Cohen and Daniel Slader, nursing home operators, were ordered to appear before the subcommittee and to supply their financial data. They were selected from a long list of homes indicted by the Better Government Association and the Chicago Tribune in their March exposé. Auditors from the U.S. General Accounting Office were assigned to aid the subcommittee with their analysis of the data supplied in compliance with its subpoenae.

Benjamin Cohen was the administrator of a 109-bed nursing home in downtown Chicago; 90 percent of his patients were on welfare. His original investment in 1967 was $40,000 on a home that cost $387,000, there being first, second, and third mortgages. Mr. Cohen had patient income of $319,000 the first year, $345,000 in 1969, and $368,000 in 1970.

In 1970, he paid himself a salary of $9,100 as administrator of the facility, and his wife $4,900 as assistant administrator. In addition to their salaries, Mr. Cohen, as 100 percent stockholder of the corporation, pocketed the difference between gross income and gross expenses. In 1970, he kept $50,292, or 13.65 percent of patient income, thus bringing in a total net income of $81,805 before taxes. In addition, the facility showed a depreciation of $31,513, bringing the total cash flow to $95,808. In 1969, he spent 67 cents per patient per day for food.

Senator Percy stated:

> So the equity, and I ask you now... because I want to make an unfair analysis here; considering the exposure is $40,000, that if everything went wrong and the mortgages, all of them could take the building over, but there is no loss beyond that; so that the investment as to equity is $40,000 and if in this 1 year $50,000 was earned, after all expense had been paid, so that the return on investment, that is equity risk, is something over 100 percent.... So you get the $31,000 cash flow and you put that against the mortgage and so the income from the Government for these patients is paying for the building simultaneously along with paying a $50,000 profit plus $13,000 or $14,000 in salaries.

Mr. Cohen responded in part:

> ...in any business there has to be profit. You don't go into it giving of your time and I am just speaking generally, and that

is the impression that people have. That is, general, but they put their investment in, they put in their time and efforts and they take the risks and I have the risk.

Daniel Slader was the administrator of a nursing home in downtown Chicago with 180 patients. Described as a skilled nursing facility, the home contained many discharged mental patients, most of whom were under 65. In the fashion of a great many homes in Illinois and Massachusetts, Mr. Slader's facility was owned by two entities. There was an operating corporation on top and a partnership on the bottom that owned the land—a classic Illinois land trust. The same four people held the entire interest in both entities. Mr. Slader and his wife each held a 25 percent interest, and a dentist, Dr. Wolski, with his wife held the remaining 50 percent.

The facility, a five-story hotel, was purchased in 1959 for $100,000. Some $40,000 in cash was put up, of which $10,000 came from Mr. Slader. By 1970, Mr. Slader's equity had grown to $250,000. In 1970, the corporation showed net profits after taxes of $51,747. Slader, his wife, and his partner paid themselves $73,500 in their capacity as officers of this corporation. In addition, the operating corporation paid a monthly rent to the partnership (again owned by the same parties) of $5,000 a month, or a total rent of $60,000 a year.

In short, the investors realized a profit of $185,248 out of total revenues of $400,000 in 1970. To this could be added $20,094 in depreciation which constituted cash flow available for operating expenses or working capital. The total profit in these terms was $205,432. In that year, Mr. Slader spent 58 cents per patient per day for food, while jails in Chicago, as Senator Adlai Stevenson pointed out, spent 64 cents a day for each inmate's food.

Mr. Slader commented:

I believe the figures are inaccurate, Senator, to begin with. I believe the net income, the real net income from this property is below what is expected in this industry. The figures haven't yet come out in the testimony.

Senator Percy:

What does the industry reasonably expect then and by what standards is it judged?

Mr. Slader:

I want to make this clear. I don't believe that the industry has established a standard but there are people who invest in nursing homes who have stated what they believe to be a reasonable return on investment, and I am merely quoting these unnamed persons, so to speak.

The impression I have is that the average investor in nursing homes expects a return of something like 15 percent to 20 percent per year on his investment in this type of enterprise.

Mr. Slader told the committee that his personal equity was in "the area of $250,000."

Senator Percy:

So that then, you would then expect that your profits should be on that, around $50,000 a year, 20 percent is it?

Mr. Slader:

Well, if we maximize it at 20 percent, yes, sir.

The mere fact that a corporation indicates losses on its tax return does not necessarily mean that no profit is being made. The subpoened records disclosed, for example, that Mr. Slader's corporation in 1962, its first year of operation as a nursing home, had a $100,000 tax loss on the basis of 41 beds. This would not be uncommon in a first year's operation, but it is to be remembered that the total purchase price of the facility was $100,000.

In that year the operating corporation paid the partnership owning the facility a rent of $72,000 on this $100,000 building! In other words, the officers of entity number one paid themselves, as entity number two, $72,000 in rent. The rent, of course, is listed on the IRS return as a business expense. The effect is not only that the corporation paid no tax for the year in question, but it also had a loss carry-forward with which to offset the income earned in succeeding years.

The Connecticut Study

In July of 1971, the Connecticut Department of Finance and Control, Budget Division, released a study of nursing home profits in that state. The report detailed an average overall return on investment of 44 percent. Excluding officers' salaries, the return on investment was 15.6 percent.

At the time when the top 500 U.S. corporations were showing a seven to eight percent rate of return, the nursing home industry, at least in Connecticut, had a minimum 15 percent rate of return. This rate of return is high as it is, but when computed before personal compensation for services, the rate of return approaches the phenomenal. It is worth noting that the returns are in line with what Mr. Slader said were industry expectations.

The Connecticut study was denounced by the industry as unfair and biased, which caused the subcommittee staff to seek the counsel of GAO auditors, who verified the validity of the accounting procedures. This same study was quoted in a confidential memo to President Nixon from then Secretary Elliot Richardson, dated July 16, 1971, which begins with the premise:

> The preponderance of informed opinion outside the industry itself contends that the present payment rates in the majority of states, especially the larger and more affluent states, are quite sufficient to support a level of services exceeding Federal minimum requirements. However, these are opinions — educated judgments — and the studies necessary to document them have not been made.

The memo continues to discuss the Connecticut study saying,

> We suggest that the situation in Connecticut is not atypical. The Connecticut licensure and inspection program is reputed to be above average.... The average Medicaid payment to nursing homes in Connecticut is $339 per month. This is close to the median for all Medicaid states, ranking 23rd in 49 jurisdictions. Thus, in Connecticut, not notably a low cost state, nursing homes [which] may be presumed to meet or exceed all Federal minimums, can realize profits averaging from 35 to 45 percent on the basis of a Medicaid payment which is equalled or exceeded by almost half the states.
>
> The dramatic influx of new capital into the nursing home industry with the advent of Medicare and Medicaid as third party payers also suggests that the economics of the industry in Connecticut are not atypical. An industry which loses money on more than half of its customers does not expand. An industry which shows above normal profit possibilities attracts capital.

The Subcommittee's 1971 Questionnaire

In an effort to obtain information from other states, the subcommittee sent questionnaires to 75 nursing homes, 25 each in three states—Massachusetts, Minnesota, and Illinois. After waiting six months from the time the original questionnaires were sent out and after three written follow-up notices reminding the operators of the subcommittee's request for information, only 21 questionnaires were received. This lack of cooperation left the committee with the decision of whether to subpoena the records of the other nursing homes or attempt to gather data some other way.

Considering the number of times the subcommittee staff heard nursing home operators contend that welfare rates were inadequate, it was almost inconceivable that they would be unwilling to share the books which would prove such contentions. But this was indeed the case. Nor was anything presented even resembling a good reason for not sharing the information. Certain nursing homes were more willing to suffer the bad publicity inherent in receiving a subpoena than they were to turn the documents over voluntarily.

Like the Senate subcommittee, the state of Michigan also had difficulty acquiring access to nursing homes' financial records, even though operators claimed that their allowed rates were not high enough. There, a struggle between the governor and the nursing home association over a few pennies in rates caused a large number of elderly to be thrown out onto the street. The following appeared in a *Detroit News* editorial on August 13, 1968:

> Last week 17 private nursing homes in Wayne County suddenly sent 34 elderly sick people to Wayne County General Hospital, with no notice to the hospital and, it appears, scant notice to their patients. The first notice the hospital says, was when two patients arrived at the door by taxicab.
>
> The hospital was not prepared. Neither were most of the patients. Though 34 came from 17 homes in two days, a spokesman for the state nursing home association said, with a straight face, that nothing was planned. He thought it was just coincidence.

Two years later the battle was still raging. An editorial by Detroit radio station WXYZ radio captures the mood: "The State wants to reclassify some patients to lower categories of care. The nursing homes say reclassification will result in a loss of income. They say their costs are too high now and their income too low. The State says simply: Prove it. Show us your books. The homes refuse and threaten eviction of the elderly."

The homes were steadfast in this refusal to let the state see their financial records. The Michigan Governor's Commission on Nursing Home Problems had to resort to tax data supplied to the Michigan Department of Treasury for the partial data it assembled for its analysis. Accordingly, one of the major conclusions of this report was that legislation be enacted which would require nursing homes to submit annual cost reports to the state government. "Regardless of the *way* facilities are reimbursed for care rendered to publicly supported patients, cost reporting is necessary to arrive at an equitable dollar value for reimbursement.... Cost reporting from all types of services largely supported by public funds will be absolutely necessary, both at operations and planning/evaluation levels."

While the subcommittee never did receive the results it asked for from the remaining nursing homes receiving its questionnaire, the GAO tabulated the 21 returns which the subcommittee did receive. Most of the homes made money. Some made a great deal of money. Return on investment quotients in excess of 100 percent were not uncommon. Specifically, only four homes lost money; the largest loss was $91,396. The largest profit was $175,000. The range of net income as a percent of gross income ranged from a low of 0.6 to a high of 20.9 percent.

The 1972 Subcommittee Study

Rather than subpoena the books and records of the remaining 54 nursing homes, Senator Moss asked the GAO to collect data on 90 nursing homes, 30 each in three states—Tennessee, Massachusetts, and Colorado. Each of these states has laws requiring administrators to file their financial information with the state. Since the information was readily available, the GAO selected a statistically valid sample. Neither the GAO nor the subcommittee looked behind these cost and financial statements to ascertain their accuracy—such accuracy was assumed. Table 5-1 shows the results.

The key figure, obviously, is the increase of average net income per home and per bed. These figures are all the more astonishing in light of the fact that 31 homes in the sample of 90 lost from $109,286 to $1. Forty-nine homes showed a profit from $0 to $50,000, seven had profits in the $50,000 to $100,000 range, and three had profits over $100,000. Average occupancy rates were 92 percent.

Table 5-1

	1969	1971	Percent Increase
Gross Income	$27 million	$36 million	
Average Gross Income per Home	$337,974	$403,586	19.4
Net Income	74,591	$1,150,033	
Average Net Income per Home	$9,357	$12,778	36.6
Gross Income per Bed	$4,245	$4,796	13.0
Net Income per Bed	$11.60	$152.00	1,166.0
Average Food Cost per Patient per Day		$1.18	

The 1972 HEW Profits Study

In October of 1971, HEW Undersecretary John Venman appeared before the subcommittee, and in response to questions concerning the Connecticut study showing 44 percent return on investment, stated that he was concerned about the possibility of excessive profits. He agreed to provide the subcommittee with a broad-based, scientific study on nursing home profits. The study data was derived from the National Center for Health Statistics in cooperation with the Census Bureau. Information concerning approximately 750 homes with 14,000 patients was obtained. In this study the average Medicare participating facility had net profits of one dollar per patient per day, while non-Medicare facilities across the nation averaged 74 cents a day profit.

The study notes that homes with high occupancy tend to have constant profits of about $1.56 per day or a profit rate of 11.1 percent per patient day. High-occupancy non-Medicare homes had profits of $1.02 a day, implying a gross sales profit rate of 10.1 percent. However, homes with low occupancy rates (below 91 percent) earned only marginal or zero profits.

The American Lutheran Church Study

Reverend John Mason, former director of Services to the Aging for the American Luthern Church (ALC) reacted sharply to costs presented by a for-profit nursing home built under one particular FHA program. In a news conference, he roundly condemned "profiteering" by some segments of the health care industry. He offered audited financial statements from ALC nonprofit homes to support his contention. The 140 ALC homes reported average costs per patient per day of $12.58 in 1972. This is contrasted with the $14.42 per patient the states paid nursing homes participating in the Medicaid program in 1972 and well below the Medicare average for that year of $32.70 per day.

Mason's study reinforces the conclusions of the confidential memo to President Nixon, "that present payment rates are quite sufficient to support a level of services exceeding Federal minimum requirements." It strengthens the implication that the possibility for large profits exists in the nursing home industry—long taken to be undisputed fact within the banking community.

The Cost of Living Council

In January of 1974, the Cost of Living Council (CLC), created by President Nixon to control inflation, filed a brief in the U.S. District Court for Washington, D.C. for the purpose of continuing its price controls on nursing homes. The CLC charged that nursing homes and their rapidly increasing costs were fueling the fires of inflation. After its detailed study, CLC concluded in its brief and supporting documents that "there is immense profitability in owning and operating nursing homes."

The Subcommittee's Study of Corporate Ownership

Immediately after Congress passed the Medicare and Medicaid legislation, prognosticators on Wall Street sensed the forthcoming expansion of nursing homes. Many operators were persuaded to "go public." Promoters argued: "The motel chains drove out the operators of roadside cabins. The grocery chains captured the retail food industry from the independents. Now the public corporations, owning multiple facilities, will take over the nursing home industry."

Major corporations such as Holiday Inn, Sheraton Inns, Quality Inns, CNA, Walter Kiddie, Cenco, INA, and Clorox entered the nursing home market hoping to share the wealth. Soon, nursing homes were the hottest issue on Wall Street. One of the high-flyers was called Four Seasons; it opened at $11 a share and was soon selling at $110 a share.

Testifying before the Subcommittee on Long Term Care, Ralph Nader asked the subcommittee to look into corporate manipulations in the nursing home field. He and others have argued that when big business takes over what has essentially been a service industry, there will be an evitable collision between the profit motive and high standards of care. This conflict is much greater than in the general operation of individual for-profit homes. In the chain operation, the importance of profit is multiplied. Investors expect yearly growth and return. This is the entire reason for chain operations — greater profits by reason of lower unit costs.

In a typical chain operation, franchises, which are a source of revenues, will be sold. It may have a subsidiary in charge of projects development. There may be yet another wholly owned subsidiary which builds the nursing homes, and yet another from which it purchases the lumber and supplies for construction. The corporation may also have a subsidiary which sells pharmaceutical supplies. With these subsidiaries, the possibility exists for charging exhorbitant amounts for construction, lumber, drugs, or whatever with the promise of repayment from Medicare and Medicaid.

In 1969, the Nixon administration sharply cut back on Medicare expenditures to nursing homes. This and the Vietnam war coupled with high inflation and high interest rates sent the stock market into a decline. Nursing home stocks tumbled. Four Seasons declared bankruptcy and stock fraud charges erupted in every direction.

In 1974, the subcommittee staff conducted a study of the financial position of the 106 major nursing home chains which had survived and were now being traded over the counter or on the New York or American Stock Exchanges. It was learned that these chains controlled roughly seven percent of U.S. nursing homes and about 18 percent of all nursing home beds. At the same time, they controlled fully one-third of the $3.26 billion paid to nursing homes in 1972.

Through its questionnaire and with the help of the Securities and Exchange Commission, the subcommittee documented the growth and profitability of these chain-controlled homes.[2] Their staggering growth rates bear out the asserted profitability of the nursing home industry, particularly if Elliot Richardson's observation is held in mind: "An industry which loses money on more than half of its customers does not expand. An industry which shows above normal profits attracts capital."

Some 80 percent of the 106 corporate chains made a profit in 1972; the occupancy rate in that year was 88 percent. The average home had 114 beds. As indicated below, the average total assets of the corporations increased by 122.6 percent, average gross revenues by 149.5 percent, and net income by 116 percent between 1969 and 1972.

Table 5-2 Increases in Nursing Home Assets/Revenues/Profits of Major U.S. Corporations (1969-1972)

Category	% Increase between 1969 and 1972*
Average Total Assets of All the Corporations	122.6%
Average Gross Revenues of All the Corporations	149.5%
Average Net Income of All the Corporations	116%
Average Assets per Home	9.8%
Average Assets per Bed	14.5%
Average Revenue per Home	23%
Average Revenue per Bed	28.3%
Average Net Income per Home	6.5%
Average Net Income per Bed	11.3%*
Average Total Assets per Corporation	84.8%
Average Total Revenue per Corporation	114.2%
Average Net Income per Corporation	85.4%

*The data in this category show an increase in net income per bed for all nursing homes in the study from $293 per bed per year in 1969 to a net income of $326 per bed per year in 1972.

In 1976, the subcommittee staff updated these statistics through another questionnaire. Preliminary computations show that from 1969 through 1975, average total revenues increased by 164 percent and net profit by 200 percent.

By comparison, the *Fortune* index for the top 500 U.S. corporations indicates they had a 66 percent increase in assets, a 95 percent increase in revenues, and a 53 percent increase in income between 1969 and 1975.

While stocks for Beverly Enterprises may be at $2.50 a share, down from a 1970 high of $44, the company has increased its profits 380 percent between 1969 and 1975—from $800,000 to $3,843,000. Likewise, Hillhaven is now selling at $6.00 a share but its income increased 196 percent from $983,726 in 1969 to $2,911,000 in 1975. Medicalodges increased 297 percent from a $109,960 to a $437,000 profit at the end of 1975.

The stocks may be low, but the revenues and the profits continue to be high.

The Moreland Act Commission

Following the disclosures of widescale fraud and abuse in nursing homes reported by the *New York Times* and later by the Subcommittee on Long Term Care, New York Governor Hugh Carey appointed a commission with extraordinary powers to investigate nursing homes in that state. Seven reports were released in early 1976. Among the commission's most important findings was the conclusion that an honest nursing home operation, in conformance with state and federal standards, could easily show a 25 percent profit or better each year. Obviously, dishonest operators can and do clear higher margins.

PROFITEERING, PENURY, AND KICKBACKS

The preceeding section dealt with what nursing home operators publicly claimed as profits. There are a million ways to cheat Medicare and Medicaid, and assuming that operators want to try a few of them, their *real* profits can be astronomical. To provide some idea of the range, one owner informed the subcommittee that he reported only 30 percent of the income he received to the Internal Revenue Service. Since there is a dearth of field audits and few prosecutions resulting from cheating the government, operators have every incentive in the world to cheat. Following are some of the more common techniques for profiteering (i.e., claiming an unreasonable profit at the expense of the patients).

Misappropriating Patients' Funds

Congress has provided that every nursing home patient on Medicaid is entitled to a $25-a-month personal spending allowance. Nursing home operators have control over these funds and are obligated by federal regulation to keep them in trust for the patients. This is one of the areas where most nursing homes fall short. After numerous complaints, Senator Moss asked the GAO to conduct a five-state audit to ascertain just how widespread the problem is. In March 1976, GAO presented its report, which concluded that *all of the 30 homes they examined* failed to safeguard patients' funds in one or several ways. GAO found shortages in patients' funds, medical supplies and services being charged to these funds, funds of deceased or transferred patients being kept by the facilities, and interest on patients' funds being kept by the facility. In one case an operator used these funds as collateral for a personal loan.

There has been only one conviction of an operator for the misuse of patients' funds. In that Seattle case, the defense attorney argued, unsuccessfully, that his client should not be convicted for "borrowing" from the patients' funds because it was the common industry practice.

Hidden Charges

Another method of profiteering involves the use of hidden charges. Families who pay for the care of their relatives may be misled into thinking that an offered monthly rate is all-inclusive. They might find out later that a raft of ancillary charges have been added. Former Congressman (now Governor) David Pryor of Arkansas printed the following schedule of such ancillary charges in the *Congressional Record*, with the following comments:

> I would call your attention to the item "Air Mattress, $45.00 per month." How many times over would a bed-ridden patient pay for this product?
>
> Here's another: "Bed Sore Care, $3.00 per day." This could well add $90.00 a month to a patient's bill.
>
> Here is "Hand feeding, $45.00 a month." Is this an honest "additional charge" for a bedridden patient who may be unable to feed himself?
>
> On the surface, this particular home bills its patients a reasonable fee — $595.00 per month for a private room — but the "extra charges" above could quickly bankrupt an unsuspecting son, daughter or patient.

Admission Sets	$ 3.50
Air Mattress	45.00 per month
Air Worms	3.50

Alcohol	.50 per pint
Aspirator	5.00 per day or use
Baby Oil	1.00
Bed Sore Care	3.00 per day
Bibs, Plastic	2.50
Bladder Irrigation Tray	1.50
Body Lotion	1.00
Catheters (Foley)	3.50
Catheterization Sets	2.00
Chest Restraints	10.00
Denture Cups	.25
Diabetic Diet	15.00 per month
Disposable Chux	.15 each
Drainage Bags and Tubing for	
Catheterization Sets	1.00
Emesis Basin	1.50
Enemas: Fleet/Oil	1.00
Foam Cushion or Ring	4.85
Guest Trays:	
Luncheon or Breakfast	1.00
Evening Meal	1.50
Hand Feeding	45.00 per month
Hand Restraints	3.00
Hypodermyclysis Set	2.00
Intravenous Set	2.00
Incontinent Care (Including Chux)	80.00 per month
Intensive Nursing Care—	
Terrace Floor	90.00 per month
Irrigation Set	1.50
Levine Tubes	2.00
Liter Cytol Urologic Irrigating Fluid	2.50 per liter
Medicated Powder	1.40
Nasal Catheters	1.00
Oxygen:	
1/4 Tank or Less	10.00
1/2 Tank	15.00
Oxygen Mask	1.00
Personal Laundry	10.00 per month
Plastic Gloves	.10
Posey Restraints	6.00
Rectal Tubes	1.00
Restraining Chair	N/C

Shampoo	1.00 per pint
Sheepskin (Synthetic)	10.00
Solutions for Clysis and I.V.'s	5.00 per bottle
Spray Deodorant	1.30
Suction Machine	25.00 per month
Suction Tube	.50
Television in Room	21.00 per room
Tissues	.25
Trapeze	15.00 per month

Supplementing Medicaid

Federal regulations prohibit charging the patient or the family any amounts over and above the Medicaid rate established by the states. However, the subcommittee has received evidence that homes charge families for ancillary charges. In other cases, families are asked to supplement the Medicaid rate if they expect their relatives to receive "first class" care. In this connection, Walter Adams, president of the Connecticut chapter of the National Council of Senior Citizens, told the subcommittee, "There are some convalescent hospitals that have three services; namely a private section; another for Medicare patients and a third for welfare patients. There are three types of meals; one for private patients, a second for Medicare patients and a third type of meal for welfare patients." A New York operator was recently convicted for telling a family that on Medicaid they could expect their mother to be placed in the dilapidated, original section of a home, but for a few dollars on the side, a bed in the new wing could be found.

A more subtle variation of the same scheme requires the family to make a "gift" or "donation" as a precondition of the nursing home's accepting a Medicaid (welfare) patient. In Miami, Florida, one administrator required the children of a patient to sign a contract which stipulated their mother was conditionally accepted until they paid an $8,500 "gift" in addition to the $900 a month for her care in the nursing home. If the children did not permanently retain the mother in the nonprofit facility, they were required by the terms of the agreement to pay a $1,000 "pledge" to the nursing home. Exhibit 5-1 is a facsimile of that contract.

Exhibit 5-1

Splendid View Nursing Home
Miami, Florida

In consideration of the charitable and philanthropic nature of SPLENDID VIEW NURSING HOME whose existence and growth is dependent in large measure upon the voluntary donations thereto by many individuals, groups, and organizations, and in consideration of the pledges, gifts and contributions thereto made by such individuals, groups and organizations,

We, John Doe and Sylvia P. Doe, hereby pledge the sum of $8,500.00 to SPLENDID VIEW NURSING HOME, Miami, Florida, the said pledge to be payable in the following manner:

Three (3) equal installments, the first to be payable 60 days after the admission of John Doe, Sr. to the SPLENDID VIEW NURS-ING HOME. This 60-day initial period constitutes a conditional admission during which John Doe, Sr. will be afforded the opportunity of determining his desire for permanent admission under the rules and regulations of the SPLENDID VIEW NURSING HOME. If, after the initial 60-day trial period, John Doe, Sr. requests permanent admission, the $8,500.00 pledge will be paid in three (3) equal yearly installments. If John Doe Sr. does not request permanent admission, a $1,000.00 pledge will be paid by the undersigned to the SPLENDID VIEW NURSING HOME.

Date _____

Witnesses_____

John Doe _____

Sylvia P. Doe _____

State of Florida⎫
County of Dade ⎬ ss:
City of Miami ⎭

On this the ____ day of _____19____ before me personally came _____ to me known and known to be the individuals described in the foregoing instrument and they duly acknowledged to me that they executed the same as their own free act and deed. _____ Notary Public

Cutting Expenses

According to sworn testimony before the subcommittee, many operators cut expenses to the point of harming patients. These operators cut back on staff, spend as little as 50 cents per patient per day for food, weigh meat on a stamp scale, serve "mock meatloaf" or breakfasts of one-half a slice of bread and coffee, refuse to buy toothbrushes, toothpaste, and toilet paper, and have only one thermometer per floor to be used both orally and rectally. There are other ways of cutting costs, such as keeping the heat down in the winter and the air conditioning off in summer, using low wattage light bulbs or not replacing burned out bulbs, doing the laundry infrequently, not repairing the physical plant, and cutting back on clean-ups or maintenance.

Following are some examples presented to the subcommittee in sworn statements from nursing home personnel.

- A nurse's aide testified:

  The administrator doled out liquid soap an ounce at a time...they rationed toilet paper and we had nothing to clean the bathtubs. The administrator told us that Dutch Cleanser was against the regulations.

- A patient offered this statement:

  They told me I would have to go get somebody else's bedpan because they didn't have one for me.... There was also no table next to my bed so that I could keep a glass of water and my eyeglasses there. The home just did not have enough equipment. That same night I wanted to wash my face and hands, so I asked for a pan and some towels. They told me I couldn't wash my hands because they didn't have any towels.

- A LPN offered this experience:

  When they serve hamburger for dinner, they have 15 pounds of hamburger for 144 patients plus the people that work there. As an example, there was a patient we called Tiny.... Before he died he always would say to me, 'Jesus Christ, I'm starving to death.' I often took food from home for him, but he was always hungry.

• An orderly gave this sworn statement:

> They reuse catheters at this home. They are supposedly cleaned and sterilized when they have been given to me to insert. However, I have found catheters that had sediment inside of them. Even though they reuse the catheters, they will charge the patients for the cost of a new one. Relatives have asked me why they are charged for a new catheter and I have to tell them that I have not used a new catheter but have put in a used one.... I am hired as an orderly but I also end up being a maintenance man, a janitor, and did general cleanup. I want to know why I am asked to carry down the garbage, to repair broken-down articles, to scrub the dayroom and clean up the urination in the hallways. It seems to me that they should have efficient maintenance men so that I can take care of the patients.

Costs Unrelated to Patient Care

Perhaps the most common method of profiteering, next to cutting back on food, staff, and other expenses, is the presentation of unauthorized costs for reimbursement by Medicare or Medicaid. All manner of personal expenses have been presented for reimbursement. A partial list of such costs which are unrelated to patient care has been compiled by Charles J. Hynes, special prosecutor for nursing homes, state of New York. Operators have asked for and received Medicare/Medicaid reimbursement for:

- Personal maids and servants
- Private residential landscaping
- Travel expenses
- Food items at levels you would not believe
- Luggage
- Works of art, including paintings by Matisse and Renoir in one instance
- Vast quantities of liquor
- Interior decorating
- Dental and medical care
- Pharmaceuticals
- Heating fuel for private residences
- Profits to investors
- Private automobile expenses
- Private pension plans
- Vacation expenses
- Real estate taxes
- Mink coats
- Personal investment stock
- Renovations to private homes
- Entertainment
- Legal fees
- Theatre tickets
- Tickets for sporting events

— Charitable contributions
— Political contributions

— High fidelity stereo
  equipment

One common abuse was to place relatives on the payroll and seek reimbursement for their salaries, even though they provided few or no services for the facility. One operator charged New York Medicaid for a $21,926 salary paid to his first wife at a time when the operator was living with his second wife in Florida. He charged New York $3,180 for domestic help in his Florida home, $10,587 for an engineer's salary (the engineer was working on a new nursing home in Florida), $29,324 for entertainment, travel, gasoline, and diesel fuel expenses, incurred on trips to Miami, Cleveland, and New York. He also charged to New York Medicaid the operational expenses for a yacht in Florida.

Other Unallowable Costs

In January of 1977, the General Accounting Office completed its review of the types of unallowable costs most commonly presented for payment by operators in four states. Following are the most recurrent.

Failure to Offset Certain Costs with Related Income. GAO found that some nursing homes were failing to offset income from beauty shops, vending machines, and investments against related expenses. GAO pointed out that if these nonpatient care items are not offset against expenses before the costs are passed on to Medicaid, the facility will be paid twice—"once as income and again as Medicaid reimbursement for the cost of the activity that produced the income."

Paper Expenses. Nonexistent invoices, or "paper" invoices submitted by a related or friendly company, have been used to justify costs which have been passed on to Medicaid. In Minnesota such phony bills were submitted by a furniture company at the request of a nursing home owner in return for the promise that he would send them a great deal of business. The phony bills, never paid, were passed on to Medicaid and generated cash for the operator. The operator was indicted and convicted of fraud in 1976.

Capital Items Expensed Rather than Capitalized. The GAO found that such capital items as permanent improvements in a building, kitchen equipment, and wheelchairs were expensed for tax purposes. In some cases, capital items were both capitalized and expensed. The result is that the facilities are reimbursed twice during the useful life of the items.

Duplicate Payments from Medicare and Medicaid. This abuse has become much less of a problem in recent years since the Medicare nursing home benefit has all but totally evaporated. But the abuse occurs often enough to deserve mention.

Collecting Payments for Patients Who Are Dead or Discharged. GAO reported in one audit of California's Medicaid nursing home program that "in 22 of the 260 cases examined, claims were paid after a recipient had died or had been discharged from the nursing home."

Trading in Real Estate

There is a heavy traffic in the buying and selling of nursing homes. The reasons for this are many and complicated, but there appear to be two primary reasons. The first involves taxes. The Internal Revenue Service allows the operator each year to deduct as depreciation an amount equal to ten percent of the value of the property he purchased. The purchase price of the nursing home becomes the basis for such depreciation; the larger the purchase price, the more that can be taken off of the operator's taxes. At the same time, if the purchase involves a minimum down payment (usually the case), most of the payments paid by the operator in the first few years will go for interest, which is deductible on the operator's taxes and also reimbursable from Medicaid.

The second reason involves the reimbursement formula for Medicare and Medicaid. The formula offers the operator a return on the investment. One way to increase the return on investment is continually to sell one home and trade it for something more expensive. One nursing home in New York was sold back and forth between related parties some eleven times in eight years. As the purchase price of the nursing home goes up, the new purchaser's equity increases and the higher and higher costs can be passed along to Medicaid. And that, after all, is the name of the game.[3]

Kickbacks

A final and pervasive method of profiteering is soliciting and receiving kickbacks. A kickback is the practice whereby a supplier is forced to pay a certain percentage of the price of nursing home supplies back to the nursing home operator for the privilege of providing supplies or services to the nursing home.

In testimony before the subcommittee in November 1976, Special Prosecutor Hynes estimated that half of the nursing homes in New

York City were involved in kickback schemes with various vendors and suppliers. The basis for his statements was an undercover investigation in which several salespeople and nursing home operators were cooperating with his office, wearing portable recording equipment. The equipment picked up the most incriminating evidence imaginable. Kickbacks between clinical laboratories and nursing homes were also documented in the course of the subcommittee's investigations in Chicago in February 1976.

Another dimension is added when the nursing home operator holds interest in a service or supply business. An October 1973 report of the National Funeral Directors Association recognized the problem, stating, "The tie which could exist between the nursing home and the funeral home whose proprietor also owns such facilities or has money invested in it is obvious."

But in most common usage, the term "kickbacks" is associated with the practice of sharing the money the government pays for nursing home drugs. The technique employed is as follows. The pharmacist presents with his drug deliveries an unitemized bill for prescriptions to the nursing home. The nursing home then "bills" each individual patient, collecting from those who pay for their own drugs and sending the rest of the bills along to the welfare department, which pays without scrutinizing it very carefully. The nursing home receives the state's check and keeps a certain percentage of it for "handling," "services rendered," or whatever.

In 1968, the Committee on Aging received a report by the attorney general of California which charged that nursing home drug kickbacks were common practice in that state and that the amount of the kickbacks ranged from 25 to 40 percent of the total price of the prescriptions delivered to the nursing home. The California legislature reacted with a statute making such kickbacks illegal.

But complaints from California continued to be received by the subcommittee. In 1970, the American Pharmaceutical Association charged flatly that pharmacists must give a kickback in order to get a nursing home account. Two years later the subcommittee staff worked closely with that association, writing and sending a questionnaire to every pharmacist in California. Some 42 percent of those who answered the questionnaire stated that they had been approached for a kickback, and another 20 percent indicated a belief that the practice was widespread. Pharmacists projected $10 million in losses in 1972 because of their failure to go along with kickbacks. The average kickback reported was 25 percent of the total Medicaid reimbursement paid the pharmacy for nursing home pharmaceuticals.

But pharmacists did not limit their response to answering the questionnaire. Many provided names of fellow pharmacists and nursing home operators alledgedly involved, others made incredible admissions about their participation in this "forced profit-sharing." A few pharmacists placed the responsibility for kickbacks on their own profession: "In order to testify, I would have to name the most important members of our association. Sorry, I am too small now." Others placed responsibility on both parties: "The ethical pharmacists are not usually approached for a percentage kickback, most are prearranged by both sides."

But most of the replies were on the other side of the ledger. One pharmacist wrote, "I'm afraid to testify. My biggest account is a nursing home. If I lost this business who will sustain me?" Another wrote, "In one pharmacy we served about 12 nursing homes. We were required to pay 25 percent to the operators of several of the homes and lost the business of three of them when we attempted to cut the kickback to 20 percent. The volume loss was in the vicinity of $5,000 a year."

Pharmacists reported that kickbacks can be in cash, usually 25 percent of total prescription charges, or a flat $5,000 a year. They can be in the form of long term credit arrangements or, in some cases, unpaid pharmacist bills. They can be in the form of rental of space in the nursing home — $1,000 a month for a closet, for example — or they can be in the form of a pharmacy bill to an individual patient, with the home keeping 25 percent of the total bill as a "collection fee." Some pharmacists supply free drugs, vitamins, and supplies, offer merchandise to employees at no charge, or deliver personal cosmetics and pharmacy needs for nursing home personnel and charge them to the home.

Other pharmacies pay the salary of certain nursing home employees who ostensibly work for the pharmacy. Still others noted that outright gifts of large quantities of green stamps, new cars, color televisions, boats, desks, and prepaid vacations to Hawaii or Europe are made. Some are required to advertise in the home's brochure at ten times normal prices. Some nursing homes have opened their own pharmacy and offer shares in the corporation to other nursing homes if they agree to use this new pharmacy. The following examples of each of these abuses are quoted directly from replies the subcommittee received.

Cash

Another means of kickback is accomplished by just sending over to the owners (Physician-owners love this one.) 20-25%

of previous month's gross or a present fee in cold cash every month. Just put eight fifty dollar bills or whatever in an envelope and hand deliver it to him or them.

Credit

One such method to which I have been personally subjected in at least a couple of instances involved very strong pressure to grant excessive credit in amounts never allowed anyone else. In each case, the operator folded, leaving me stuck with an uncollectable bill of one to two thousand dollars each time.

You might not consider this to be a 'kickback'. I do, for its origins, cause and effect were precisely the same as in the more formal instances you might have in mind.

Renting Space

Both places wanted me to *rent* a complete room in ECF plus supplying their own personal needs. This (at that time) was about $1100-1200/month with an estimated percent to volume of about 20-25%. The pharmacy that had the "*contract*" was renting a linen closet for $700/month "storage." The home owner also wanted me to explore with him the setting up of a company to supply these rest homes (he had 2 and 1 in the planning stage) since if the supply costs were high they would do better since they were on a cost-plus percentage with the health agencies.

Supplies

I was requested to supply the nursing home with such things as mineral oil, aspirin, gauze pads, tape, etc., free of charge. These were things that the nursing home was being paid to supply in the daily rates set by the state.

a) I was also requested to mail out prescriptions for drugs that were not used, but instead I was asked to supply things that the nursing home was supposed to supply. These were to be charged to welfare. Example: make out a prescription for antibiotic and charge to welfare but instead send to the patient a Posey belt (restraining device).

b) I was approached by an administrator of a convalescent hospital on supplying prescriptions and supplies to that facility, the only IF, that I would charge all of her cosmetics and pharmacy needs to the hospital, indicating that these were Drug Store supplies for the facility.

"Hiring" Nursing Home Employees for the Pharmacy

Kickbacks demands are in various forms, not necessarily cash rebates. Two examples are: the supplying of certain drugs, vitamins, and supplies at NO CHARGE to the ECF. Paying the monthly salary of a full-time employee whose sole duty is to tell the pharmacy whether the patient is a Medi-Cal, Medicare, or private patient in the ECF, thus ostensibly working as an employee of the pharmacy, but in reality working for the ECF.

Trading Stamps

Kickbacks in this area are more subtle. For example, green stamps, advertising in facilities' promotional brochures at 10 times the normal prices.

Color TVs & Boat

I have no real proof of kickbacks on a specific situation as far as cash is concerned—however, I do know that on the Xmas of one year, color TVs were delivered and paid for by one of the stores—also, the following year a boat was given—also, massive amounts of trading stamps are sent to the facility.

Prepaid Vacations

In this area the "kickback" is in the form of personal gratitude such as prepaid trips to Hawaii, Japan, a new desk, free use of a ski cabin, beach house, or other valuable usage.

Advertising

Because of my refusal to "buy advertising space" in their monthly nursing home newsletter (a three page affair) priced at $124 per month (my rate computed at 10% of Medi-Cal charges and 15% of private patient charges), I was dropped as the pharmacy to provide services. Whether I buy advertising space or slip them the money in cash under the table, it is still graft and I certainly hope you're able to stem this horrible practice. I wrestled with my conscience as to whether I should suffer the $15,000 a year loss or whether I should "make up the difference" on charges for any new prescription for the private patients that would be reimbursed under extended care Medicare funds. You would be absolutely amazed at the amount of government money which is being sopped up by these "extra billings."

Automobile Leasing

Another approach is that of auto leasing for the home's administrator. May be given him as a fringe benefit of his job by the owners. All kinds of things can be worked out by the leasing company whereby it is almost completely tax deductible. Most pharmacies have delivery cars; usually small and compact cars with low monthly leasing fees. Now, a new Mark III leases for $225.00/month and a VW delivery car for $50.00 monthly. The leasing agency writes up any kind of lease it wishes; it can lease the Mark III to the rest home owners for $75.00 per month and charge the Pharmacy $200.00 per month for the VW. Everybody is happy. IRS cares not because somebody is going to write off the car as expense anyway, no cash has been lifted from the Pharmacy so no books have to be juggled, and you get the business.

Purchasing Stock or Shares in the Facility

a) Owners of nursing homes in our area have joined forces and opened Pharmacies which only service nursing homes. They then offer interest in their Pharmacy to other nursing home operators if they will use the Pharmacy.

b) One nursing home in our area approached Drug Stores in our area as to amount of kickback they would give to get the drug business. It was given to one drugstore. This went on for sometime. Then the manager (a Circuit Court Judge) asked the Drug Store supplying drugs to nursing homes to buy stock in said nursing home for the business. This he wouldn't do and business was taken away and given to a Drug Store that did. The amount of stock in Corp. was $5,000.00.

Many pharmacists wrote of their serious concern about the conflict of interest presented when the ownership of the pharmacy and the nursing home overlap. This arrangement increases the nursing home's ability to manipulate prescriptions to bilk the government and their ability to cover up mistakes.

Another reason I have never pursued nursing home accounts is because they are always having drug problems as most of them are operating without pharmaceutical assistance and often request drugs to cover up for some they have borrowed from another patient. They have a number of reasons for requesting drugs early and an investigtion will show that many laws are being violated daily and I don't intend to practice in this manner.

Several pharmacists wrote that the inadequate rates paid by nursing homes led them to try to make a profit in any quarter. Many also felt that the reimbursement formula for welfare medications was too low, stating that the necessity to pay kickbacks leads the pharmacist to many shortcuts. As an illustration, one pharmacist noted that a prescription might cost $4.50 plus a fee of $2.30. This was the most welfare would allow. Thus, the total price of the prescription would be $6.80, and with a 25 percent kickback of $1.70, only 60 cents would be left over for profit, salary, rent, etc. Accordingly, some of the pharmacists admitted:

1. Billing welfare for nonexistent prescriptions
2. Supplying outdated drugs or drugs of questionable value
3. Supplying stolen drugs which they have purchased or supplying discarded drugs (those belonging to dead or discharged patients);
4. Supplying drug samples which they have received free
5. Supplying generic drugs and charging the state for brand name drugs
6. Using a particular line of drugs because the manufacturer has a price list where every item is listed at a higher price than is actually charged. By using such products, the pharmacist can charge the state more and make a higher profit.

Nursing home operators are, of course, defensive. A questionnaire to all 2,050 administrators in California brought 619 returns. Some 484, or 78 percent, stated that they had never offered or accepted a kickback. Few volunteered comments. Those who did emphasized that public assistance rates were too low and went to pains to distinguish a kickback or other unearned and undisclosed consideration from "earned discounts." They emphasized that they earned discounts because of their quantity buying and because of the services they performed for the pharmacist.

Despite these denials, a few things are certain. First, the profit in drugs supplied to the nursing home is being shared. Pharmacists claim they are unwilling partners, that they are the victims of extortion. Nursing home operators allege that the discounts are voluntarily given by the pharmacists.

Second, the cost of drugs to private paying patients and to the taxpayer is being inflated. Pharmacists say that the pressure of kickbacks or discounts makes them try to get as high a price for their drugs as they can, whether the party paying is the state, the federal government, or the individual. One pharmacist wrote that an item which cost $1.79 in the pharmacy was priced $7.95 to the nursing home patient. Subcommittee files reflect many such examples, including one in which the patient's drug bill for the same medications tripled when the patient entered a nursing home.

Third, because the practice of kickbacks is widespread, some pharmacists are resorting to unethical methods to lower their costs, such as charging the government for nonexistent drugs, reusing discarded drugs, or supplying generic drugs at name-brand prices, old or ineffective drugs, samples which they have received for free, or stolen drugs.

Congress enacted a statute in October 1972, which made offering or accepting a kickback a crime punishable by a year in jail and a maximum $10,000 fine. Unfortunately, administrative regulations defining the law have yet to be issued by HEW. Consequently, existing fraud statutes are of limited use because, according to most legal scholars, fraud under their terms is difficult to prove. Not unsurprisingly, the subcommittee's follow-up questionnaire, received in January 1974, indicates that kickbacks are still widespread and that the intervening statute has had little effect.

In November of 1976, Samuel K. Skinner, United States attorney, northern district of Illinois obtained the first convictions under the 1972 federal law. Investigations were also underway in Wisconsin. Special Prosecutor Hynes had indicted 42 vendors with the promise that perhaps another 50 indictments would follow. The state of Florida conducted its own investigation, finding nursing home pharmacy kickbacks widespread in that state. And, in California, which has received intensive scrutiny, the same pattern of fraud and abuse continues virtually unchecked. Testifying before the subcommittee, Charles Brown, president of the California Pharmaceutical Association, estimated that 40 percent of the pharmacists in his state still pay kickbacks or rebates.

It is clear that while the subject of kickbacks is receiving increasing attention in a few states, there is nothing like the serious effort at investigation and prosecution which is needed. A total of only 20 Medicare or Medicaid kickback cases have been successfully prosecuted by the states or the federal government since these programs began in 1966.

Conclusions

After this intensive analysis, a few conclusions are supportable:

1. In the words of John Twiname, former administrator of the Cost of Living Council, in a brief filed in U.S. District Court in January 1974, "There is immense profitability in owning and operating nursing homes."
2. The nursing home business is particularly lucrative for large nursing home chains whose gross assets, total revenues, and net profits have increased dramatically between 1969 and the present.
3. Nursing home ownership is anything but public knowledge. By virtue of interlocking ownership officers, and directors, small groups of individuals are able to control incredible numbers of nursing homes. Such informal chains remain hidden from the public view.
4. The final line on the balance sheet is not the total answer to the profitability of nursing homes. Goals and expectations differ. Some are trying to minimize equity and "milk" their operations. Most seek to minimize their tax liability under the Internal Revenue Code and pay as little as possible.
5. In an effort to pay as little as possible in taxes, many chains engage tax planners with the goal of showing approximately a 5 percent return (profit) on gross sales. This objective can be reached by reinvesting as much as possible in new construction or the purchase of existing facilities. Corporations employ many techniques to split income or convert potential profits into increased equity. Some of these techniques include the use of wholly owned subsidiaries which deal with the parent company, the continuous turnover of property for purpose of accelerating depreciation write-offs, sale and leaseback operations, inflated rents and compensations paid to officers of the corporation, or other less than arm's-length transactions.
6. There is a need for better data on nursing home profits and for tighter controls such as a uniform chart of accounts and the requirement that all nursing homes receiving federal funds file CPA-audited financial statements. It is doubtful that the industry will volunteer information about profits, having resisted every effort in the past. This points to the need for legislation to ensure the taxpayers, who pay more than half of the nursing home bill, that appropriate use is being made of their tax dollars.
7. Beyond the profits which can be made inside the law, there are untold riches to be made by the unscrupulous who would subordinate

patient care to profits. Unfortunately, there are all too many operators who have yielded to the temptation to join this unwholesome geriatric gold rush.

8. Two of the most prevalent ways to cheat is to misappropriate the patients' personal funds and to solicit kickbacks from vendors and suppliers. There is evidence that kickbacks are widespread; vendors contend they must pay them if they hope to gain nursing homes' business.

Chapter 6
Nursing Homes: New Depositories for the Mentally Impaired

Amos Johnson was born in Chicago on the same day as the 1903 Iroquois Theatre fire, which claimed 566 lives. It was an ominous beginning for Amos, whose entire life was a tragedy. He had been born of reluctant parents who abandoned him on the steps of a Catholic church soon after they learned of his congenital deformity. He had the priest and the nuns to thank for his very survival. Despite laborious instructions from these saintly tutors, Amos never completely mastered the puzzle of connected speech.

In the bars of Chicago's south side, where he earned his keep by mopping the floors, he was known as "crazy Amos." Cruel patrons made fun of his huge head; they pitched pennies into the spitoon and roared with laughter as he went diving after them. To this dehumanizing charade, and to other games that some people play with dogs, Amos responded with the same generous and apparently permanent smile.

Something happened on that winter night in 1929, but no one was exactly sure what. Some say that Amos tried to disembowel a man named "Muzzy" with a meat clever in the kitchen of a speakeasy. Others deny this. "Muzzy" apparently was unharmed because only Amos went to the hopsital—Chicago State Mental Hospital.

After 40 years in the institution, someone decided that he and the rest of his colleagues in the geriatric ward of the hospital no longer constituted a danger to themselves or to the community. So Amos and many of his friends were released to nursing homes and old hotels in an area known as "Uptown" in Chicago. This precipitous transfer of hundreds of elderly was justified as "returning them to the community."

Amos did not fare well in the nursing home. The many days of enforced idleness left him with legs and feet swollen to twice their size.

103

Inevitably, bed sores developed. The one on his right leg got progressively worse, even though he did get intermittent treatment for it. Gangrene developed, and there was no choice but to amputate the leg at mid-thigh. On his return to the nursing home, his appetite and the smile were gone. Today he lies in bed or sits in a wheelchair and stares.

But Amos is not alone. He has hundreds and thousands of counterparts in every state of the union. All of them are victims of the latest swing of the fiscal pendulum. In an effort to preserve scarce state dollars and replace them with federal dollars, every state has embarked on an ambitious program to empty out their state mental hospitals and place people in nursing homes and other smaller community-based facilities, which traditionally have been ill-prepared to deal with the mentally impaired aged.

This trend has been evident in some states for several years. For example, in California there were 12,000 aged in state mental hospitals in 1959, but only 4,129 remained at the end of 1969. But it has only been in the past six years that this trend has accelerated into a national phenomenon.

California again helps to document the sharp and escalating trend. The number of aged in that state's hospitals dropped 86 percent between 1969 and 1974, when only 578 remained institutionalized. Massachusetts reduced its aged patient population by 87 percent, from 8,000 to 1,050; Illinois from 7,263 to 1,744. Wisconsin showed a 99 percent reduction, from 4,616 elderly patients in 1969 to 96 at the end of 1974.

These examples are merely illustrative of the national trend. In these same five years, the number of inpatients in state mental hospitals dropped 44 percent, from 427,799 to 327,692. At the same time, there was a national 56 percent reduction in the number of elderly inmates (from 135,322 to 59,685). Table 6.1 provides state-by-state totals.

IMPETUS FOR THE EXODUS

Why patients are being transferred in such tremendous numbers is superficially a mix of four factors: humanitarianism, cost, the impact of recent court decisions, and the enactment of the Supplementary Security Income Program by Congress. As indicated, a closer analysis reveals that monetary concerns are the overriding consideration.

Table 6—1 Number of Inpatients in State Mental Hospitals, 1969, 1973, and 1974, and Number Over Age 65 by State

State	Total inpatients			Percentage of decrease (or increase)		Total inpatients over age 65		
	1969	1973	1974	1969–74	1973–74	1969	1973	1974
Alabama	7,601	3,810	3,067	—60	—20.0	2,646	1,197	639
Alaska	674	831	148	—78	—83.0	27	11	0
Arizona	1,141	659	655	—43	—1.0	384	179	116
Arkansas	1,460	1,247	474	—68	—62.0	311	416	491
California	16,116	7,011	6,476	—60	—8.0	4,129	997	573
Colorado	10,317	11,952	5,652	—45	—53.0	1,250	1,379	614
Connecticut	6,068	3,892	3,597	—41	—8.0	1,611	601	568
Delaware	1,140	944	966	—15	+2.3	408	380	410
District of Columbia	5,111	2,994	2,708	—47	—10.0	2,058	1,161	1,077
Florida	9,562	8,170	6,385	—33	—22.0	3,952	3,241	1,966
Georgia	7,653	6,480	7,446	—3	+15.0	2,207	1,678	1,040
Hawaii	581	250	297	—49	+18.0	182	52	92
Idaho	527	232	207	—61	—11.0	300	100	46
Illinois	28,233	15,703	14,179	—50	—10.0	7,263	2,065	1,744
Indiana	16,703	12,866	7,735	—54	—40.0	4,209	2,783	1,248
Iowa	2,230	2,954	991	—56	—66.0	1,742	431	132
Kansas	5,592	5,961	1,298	—77	—78.0	1,175	982	114
Kentucky	3,479	1,199	1,956	—44	+63.0	873	412	390
Louisiana	4,676	3,327	2,851	—39	—14.0	553	349	255
Maine	2,726	1,249	1,480	—46	+18.0	1,072	463	442
Maryland	7,161	5,950	4,968	—31	—17.0	2,387	1,983	1,469
Massachusetts	21,000	7,500	11,688	—44	+55.0	8,000	2,300	1,050
Michigan	12,293	6,865	5,922	—52	—14.0	2,890	1,358	1,119
Minnesota	3,792	2,710	5,584	+47	+106.0	785	574	478
Mississippi	5,955	5,627	4,107	—31	—27.0	2,567	2,272	865
Missouri	7,496	5,210	4,054	—46	—22.0	2,587	1,439	807
Montana	1,376	1,104	1,057	—23	—4.0	500	453	139
Nebraska	1,685	765	2,815	+67	+267.0	382	70	208
Nevada	439	367	264	—40	—28.0	78	77	19
New Hampshire	2,074	1,446	1,306	—37	—10.0	966	672	472
New Jersey	22,857	21,616	10,695	—53	—51.0	6,563	4,981	3,680
New Mexico	700	400	337	—52	—16.0	168	61	86
New York	70,765	44,042	39,770	—44	—10.0	28,400	19,642	17,681
North Carolina	22,507	20,010	4,829	—79	—76.0	3,824	4,188	1,347
North Dakota	1,208	644	642	—47	—.5	360	200	146
Ohio	16,934	16,726	9,793	—42	—42.0	4,752	3,155	2,850
Oklahoma	3,854	2,702	2,281	—41	—16.0	713	552	507
Oregon	2,260	2,340	2,191	—4	—4.6	710	730	319
Pennsylvania	27,536	18,235	16,307	—41	—11.0	8,360	5,811	5,597
Puerto Rico	(1)	1,154	995	(1)	—14.0	(1)	129	166
Rhode Island	1,881	1,845	3,456	+84	+87.0	610	687	660
South Carolina	5,805	5,484	4,330	—25	—20.0	1,872	2,161	1,224
South Dakota	1,229	860	690	—44	—20.0	711	425	194
Tennessee	6,713	4,584	4,562	—32	—.5	1,807	1,353	1,357
Texas	14,253	9,048	8,588	—40	—5.0	5,464	2,876	1,447
Utah	1,284	823	897	—30	+9.0	209	80	96
Vermont	1,079	582	475	—56	—18.0	455	182	110
Virginia	11,338	7,740	6,072	—46	—22.0	4,100	2,700	2,614
Washington	4,252	3,738	4,286	+1	+14.5	722	430	349
West Virginia	3,950	3,507	2,869	—27	—18.0	1,194	1,206	782
Wisconsin	10,908	7,574	1,691	—84	—78.0	4,616	3,222	96
Wyoming	453	304	303	—33	....	160	95	60
Total	427,799	304,233	237,691			135,322	84,959	59,685

[1] 1969 figures for Puerto Rico not available.

Source: Committee questionnaire.

Humanitarianism

The first reason for such transfers is humanitarianism. It is the simple truth that many elderly were in asylums not because of their need for treatment but because they had no place else to go. Startling examples have been provided of people who have been committed, apparently for the singular reason that no one could understand their native language. In the same vein are numerous studies indicating that many supposedly mentally ill patients were really physically ill. Strokes or toxic confusions, for example, mimic psychotic symptoms. It was argued that these individuals who did not really belong in a mental hospital could and should be returned to the community. The same was suggested for those who had been residents of state hospitals many years and were now "burned out"—a term signifying that they were no longer of potential harm to themselves or others.

The Impact of Recent Court Decisions

A second factor which has fueled the movement of patients from state hospitals to other facilities is the impact of recent court decisions by various federal courts and most recently by the Supreme Court. In the first such influential ruling, a federal judge in Alabama held that individuals committed to state hopsitals against their will and for treatment had a constitutional right to such treatment or they had to be released.

The celebrated Supreme Court case, *O'Conner v. Donaldson*, had a similar outcome. The Court held that a state cannot constitutionally confine a non-dangerous individual who is capable of surviving safely in freedom by himself or with the help of willing and responsible family members and friends without offering treatment.

Another equally far-reaching decision came late in 1973 from the U.S. District Court in Washington, D.C. The case involved a man who had been committed to a mental institution for some 33 years where he had worked 11 hours a day, five days a week, and only nine and a half hours a day the other two days of the week, getting two days off a month and about ten dollars compensation. The Court ruled that where the state institution receives any consequential economic benefit from the employment of patients, it must pay these patients an appropriate competitive rate.

The message to the states is an economic one: You must provide treatment for inmates or release them, and if you make them work, you have to pay them a fair wage. Given the choice, most states have taken the least expensive option of releasing patients.

Cost

Cost is undoubtedly the primary reason for the transfer of thousands of patients from state hospitals to nursing homes and other facilities. The average national cost of keeping a patient in a state mental institution is presently estimated at about $1,000 a month or $12,000 a year. Such costs can be a great deal higher. For example, Gardner State Hospital in Massachusetts estimates a cost of $16,000 a year. In St. Elizabeth's Hospital, Washington, D.C., the average cost per patient is now $24,000 a year.

It should be clear that given the strain on many state budgets, there has been tremendous pressure to move patients into nursing homes, boarding homes, and old hotels. The advantage to the state is even greater than it appears. Typically, states must assume 100 percent of their mental hospital costs. If patients can be released and added to the state's welfare rolls (including Medicaid) the federal government will then pay at least half of the cost. If the state release the patients unconditionally and maintains the fiction that they are simply indigent elderly, the federal government will pay 100 percent of the cost through the new Supplementary Security Income program.

Supplementary Security Income (SSI)

In 1972, Congress created the first 100 percent federal welfare program, called Supplementary Security Income (SSI). It was an attempt to provide a minimum floor under the incomes of the aged poor. Today they receive $157 a month from the federal government in the form of gold-colored checks sent out by the Social Security Administration.

SSI is a cash grant program. The checks can be paid only to individuals, not to nursing homes. In fact, a specific prohibition was added barring SSI funds to individuals in public institutions (defined to include mental hospitals and nursing homes). But the attraction of federal money proved to be too great. In direct violation of the law, many states are using SSI funds to pay for keeping the aged in nursing homes. Even worse, the states are moving patients into unlicensed, privately owned boarding homes to make them eligible for SSI.

The cost incentives for the states are tremendous. For every individual moved from a state hospital to a boarding home, the average state's budget will be richer by the sum of $1,157 a month. The state saves the $1,000 a month in state money that it would ordinarily spend to keep the individual in a mental hospital; plus, it gains $157 a month, the amount of the federal SSI payment which goes to keep the inmate in a boarding home or old hotel.

CONSEQUENCES

It should be obvious at the outset that the consequences of the mass transfer of the infirm and impaired elderly can be severe. Indeed, investigations by the Subcommittee on Long Term Care confirm that every transfer poses significant dangers for the institutionalized elderly:

- Patients often are being discharged wholesale and indiscriminately. There is virtually no screening procedure to decide who are proper candidates for discharge.
- There are high incidents of mortality and morbidity associated with such transfers.
- There is no follow-up to determine if patients are properly placed in their new facilities.
- Nursing homes, boarding homes, or shelter care facilities are ill-equipped to handle these patients. It is not only that there are no psychiatric services available and no plans to rehabilitate patients. Dangers are also present when discharged mental patients are mixed with those who are physically ill; the effect is to reduce all patients in the home to the lowest common denominator. Put another way, individuals tend to reflect their environment and the "normal elderly" soon manifest the behavioral patterns of the disturbed patients they see around them.
- There are few, if any, recreational services or activity programs in the smaller community-based facilities.
- While most states have standards for nursing homes, few have any standards for boarding homes. Consequently, abominable conditions exist in some homes where patients are now being supported by federal Supplementary Security Income.
- There is a heavy, and perhaps unwise, use of drugs to help manage patients and make up for the fact that these facilities are badly understaffed.
- Many states have given complete and final discharges to individuals placing them together in certain areas of our cities, which have become instant "geriatric or psychiatric ghettos." For example, 13,000 patients were discharged from Illinois state

hospitals into an area called "Uptown" in Chicago. In Washington, D.C., hundreds of patients will be found near Ontario Road, NW.

The best way to demonstrate graphically the consequences both to the elderly and to the society of an influx of hundreds of former mental patients is to take one state as a case study. In this case, Illinois provides the example:

In March of 1969, legislation popularly known as the Copeland bills was proposed before the Illinois state legislature. The bills proposed:

1. removing the elderly from the state's definition of mental illness;
2. requiring the state to make an immediate evaluation of all patients admitted prior to July 1, 1964, to determine the possibility of their receiving care outside the hospital;
3. establishing screening procedures to keep new admissions down and vesting authority in the Department of Mental Health to place discharged individuals "in a suitable family home or such other facility as the Department may consider desirable."

In May, Governor Richard B. Ogilvie gave the bills his enthusiastic support and announced the state's intention to move 7,000 senior citizens out of mental institutions into nursing homes and shelter care facilities within a year and a half. These bills were signed into law in September 1969, and a press release from the governor's office began: 10,000 ELDERLY PATIENTS TO LEAVE STATE MENTAL HOSPITALS. The release quotes the governor as saying that more than 10,000 elderly citizens were living in mental hospitals—not because they were mentally ill, but simply because they had no place else to go.

Despite assurances that proper testing would be undertaken to decide who were proper candidates for discharge and that follow-up care would be provided by the Department of Mental Health to ease the return of these individuals to the community, many Chicago officials were skeptical. In July 1970, Robert Ahrens, director of the Division of Senior Citizens in Chicago wrote to the editor of the *Chicago Tribune:*

> The chief reason for placement of the elderly in state mental hospitals has been that adequate alternative community facilities were not available. They are still not available. The problem will not be resolved, nor is it fair to the elderly simply to move them around and have many small warehouses take the place of the large ones.

To support his statement, Mr. Ahrens offered a May 1970, report prepared by his office which detailed the lack of appropriate facilities to house the mentally impaired, the lack of trained personnel, and the lack of activities and supportive services to meet their needs in nursing homes.

In March of 1971, the *Chicago Tribune* and the Better Government Association (BGA) conducted their survey of nursing home conditions in Chicago. They concluded that nursing homes in Chicago were "warehouses for the dying." They cited shocking conditions, poor care, and profiteering. As a result, the subcommittee requested that the investigators work with the staff to widen the investigation of nursing homes to the entire state of Illinois. The investigators testifying at the subcommittee hearings on April 2 and 3, 1971, concluded that the transfer program had contributed to the wretched conditions in Illinois nursing homes.

Myrtle Merritt and Dr. Collette Rasmussen of the Cook County Department of Health confirmed this conclusion. With respect to one new nursing home, they testified:

> This home has almost a double file, considering its length of service. We have many, many complaints on them.
>
> It is phenomenal in its infestation with roaches. The smell on the patient floors, which are the second and third floors, is nauseating.
>
> The home itself, very shortly after it opened, was filled with busloads of conditionally discharged mental health patients all of whom now are permanent discharges; none of whom appear to be getting rehabilitation in any way.
>
> Now what is distressing to me is that we have mentally retarded people here, although they don't seem to be threatening in any way. I know that many of them at least by face and a few of them by name because I have been there that often and the patients they have and the bedrooms that they stay in are just unbelievable.

Another of the homes indicted by the investigators at the hearings was the Carver Nursing Home in Springfield, Illinois. State Department of Health inspection reports related abominable conditions, including one patient covered with bedsores from the waist down. The bedsores on the hips which were the size of grapefruits and so deep the bones could be seen. A little more than a year after the subcommittee's hearing, a fire at this nursing home claimed the lives of ten elderly.

There were 42 patients in the home at the time; 14 were discharged mental patients. Although the final cause of the fire probably never will be known, some investigators believe that the fire was started by one of the discharged mental patients.

At the subcommittee hearings in Chicago, City Health Commissioner Dr. Murray C. Brown reinforced other testimony, strongly asserting a clear relationship between the shocking conditions in Chicago nursing homes and the state's effort to remove patients from state mental hospitals: "We believe that the deterioration of facilities and care in Chicago nursing homes is directly related to the aforementioned policy changes made in 1969 by the Illinois State Legislature, the Governor, and the State Department of Mental Health."

Dr. Jack Weinberg was also critical of the state's program. As clinical director of the Illinois State Psychiatric Association, he was given the job of transferring the proposed 10,000 elderly, but quickly resigned the position when his plan to release people on a case-by-case basis was overruled. At the hearings, he related a bribe offer of $100 a head for every mental patient he would place in various nursing homes, which he rejected indignantly.

In March 1972, the BGA, with the *Chicago Sun-Times* and WLS-TV, Channel 7, Chicago's ABC-TV affiliate, conducted an investigation into the transfer of the 13,000 individuals from state hospitals into nursing and shelter care homes. They concluded that patients were being discharged "wholesale and indiscriminately" and that the principal motive was economic, since it cost the state about $1,000 a month on the average to care for patients in mental hospitals, and $300 or less in boarding homes. They reported wretched conditions, poor food, poor care, indiscriminate tranqulization, and other related abuses.

In September of 1975, J. Terrance Brunner, executive director of the BGA, testified before the subcommittee about their follow-up investigation:

> We found conditions in the homes to be substantially the same. Cosmetic changes have occurred. Walls that were covered with chipped plaster three years ago are adorned with colorful posters and nicely printed meal schedules.... But the basic problems remain: the privately owned facilities lack trained personnel, many residents are continuously oversedated, and there is no real attempt to accomplish the primary mission of integrating the residents into the life of the surrounding community.

Despite the publicity that surrounded the findings of BGA, *Sun-Times*, and Channel 7 as well as the recent nationwide publicity concerning private shelter care homes, the state's policy of shifting its responsibility to ill-equipped private homes and unprepared local communities continues. And it continues when the state's own statistics and reports present convincing evidence that the policy is a disaster.

Mr. Brunner's conclusion was given greater weight by the investigation into the deaths of seven patients at the Illinois Extended Care Center, a for-profit nursing home in Rockford, Illinois. The inquiry was conducted by the Illinois Legislative Investigating Commission, which asserted that five of the seven deaths were "avoidable," charging that negligence on the part of the nursing staff was a major factor in the deaths. "Insufficient staff observation and treatment, unacceptable and unprofessional attitudes, general irresponsible nursing performances were the rule rather than the exception." The commission's report describes one of the dead:

> William Redford, 73 years of age, died on October 24, 1973 from "broncho-pneumonia," after being placed at the Illinois Extended Care Center for a period of 22 days. The severely mentally retarded Redford received inadequate and unresponsive nursing care and treatment. He continually exhibited physical problems which either went unheeded or unattended to by the facility's nursing staff. These problems culminated in Redford's death.
>
> Redford's death raised serious questions. There was little, if any, justification for the Illinois Department of Mental Health and Developmental Disabilities to place a 73-year old person with over 57 years of institutionalization in the Illinois Extended Care Center. Redford's residency at IECC was devoid of any aftercare supervision by Department personnel.

If all of this were not bad enough, Illinois authorities soon discovered that 17 patients had died in 17 months at the All Seasons Nursing Home in Waukeegan, Illinois. State inspection reports disclosed that nurses pleaded with the state to stop sending the mentally impaired to this nursing home, which was reportedly understaffed and whose few employees had little training in how to take care of discharged inmates. Dr. Richard Blanton, director of developmental disabilities, state of Illinois, said the reports of inadequate care at the facility had gone ignored by state officials.

I don't understand how they were maintaining their license. The thing of it is, we were getting reports that it was a marginal facility as far back as July of 1973.

Illinois and Lake County Inspection records show that 88 profoundly retarded patients were found in a state of confusion. Everyone in the unit was wet, covered with feces, and caked food. Many were lying naked. Investigators found one female patient infested with maggots.

At the hearings conducted by the subcommittee, Dr. Weinberg placed this entire problem in perspective. He characterized the state's discharge program as "good theory — bad execution." He argued that if supportive and protective services were available, the mentally impaired should be in the community, but such services are not available. He continued:

I believe further that many of our mental institutions, even though some of them may be snake pits, are better places than some of the nursing homes in view of the fact that they at least have such necessary items of care as 24-hour coverage by a nurse, a fire alarm system and the food in the State hospitals is nutritionally adequate; and some facilities for some minimal activities is also present in most mental institutions of the States.

The Illinois experience is not unique, and Dr. Weinberg is not alone in his views. Similar statements have been made by psychiatrist Dr. Robert Butler, director of the National Institute on Aging, and by Dr. Leonard Gottesman of the Philadelphia Geriatrics Center. Gottesman says that the trend to move patients from state hospitals in nursing homes "is potentially dangerous because there are no real plans for improving the patients' care in community nursing homes."

Dr. George Warner points out that 55 to 80 percent of the patients in nursing homes have some degree of mental impairment. He says many quickly receive the label of "senility," which, to the staff, means the patient is "hopeless" and can be ignored. He asserts that individuals with mental impairment are the most poorly served in today's nursing homes. He charges the lack of physician leadership and management results in the "overutilization of depressant-stimulant drugs, physical restraints or both."[1]

The fact that such a large number of patients with mental disabilities have been consigned to nursing homes is a realization of Margaret Blenkner's worst fears. Years ago she had written:

> Nursing homes have little to do with meeting the mental health needs of the aged now and I hope they will have even less in the future. Nursing homes are less capable of meeting the mental health needs of their residents than the institutions from which many of the mentally ill have been transferred. A not inconsiderable share of the mental health problems of nursing home patients arise out of their being there.[1]

Margaret Blenkner implies what English expert Dr. Lionel Z. Cousin claims to be fact. He suggests that when elderly with mental deterioration are placed in a facility housing the infirm elderly the effect is to reduce the patient population to the lowest common denominator. He said: "very often the confused elderly pick up their confusion, their first symptoms of violence and agitation, from the anxious, occasionally violent environment."

Dr. Charles Kramer, of Chicago, Illinois, noted psychiatrist and president of the Kramer Foundation, agrees that trying to treat individuals having a combination of physical and psychological impairment can be a devastating problem. He adds: "Most of my psychiatrist friends shy away from this field. That means that (in nursing homes) a girl with only a high school education may be dealing every day with serious psychological problems, with serious interpersonal relationship problems, and she is expected to manage, not only these, but severe physical disability in patients as well."

Most of these experts agree with Dr. Kramer that the absence of trained personnel in nursing homes is the key to the poor past performance. They also agree that it is the presence of trained personnel that causes the cost of treatment in a state mental hospital to reach levels of $24,000 a year and beyond. Consequently, if nursing homes were staffed at hospital levels they might likely be as costly as state hospitals. Indeed, costs in nursing homes may even be higher. Should this happen, it is likely that Amos Johnson and his surviving friends would once again be carted up and transported back to state hospitals.

Dr. Karl Menninger, founder of the Menninger Foundation, told the subcommittee, "the saddest part of all this is the fact that recovery is possible even with the most severely impaired, psychotic and hopeless patients if they are approached with sensitive and highly motivated treatment." He told of 88 patients in the geriatric ward of the Topeka State Hospital:

> They were hopeless psychotics. Many had been there over 10 years; one had been there 58 years. When approached by a team of cheerful doctors, nurses and social workers wherein each patient became the focus of attention, they showed remarkable improvement. As the results of new programs, activities and therapies, only 9 of the 88 patients were still bedfast at the end of the year. Only six were still incontinent. Five had died. Twelve had gone to live with their families. Six had gone to live with themselves, and four had found comfortable provisions outside the hospital. Four of the original 88 were now gainfully employed and self-supporting.

If these results can be achieved among the most helpless and hopeless patients in the geriatric ward of a Kansas hospital, then it is obvious that thousands of others on the financial merry-go-round could and should be helped.

Chapter 7

No Vacancy for Minority Groups

Both age and illness are a jeopardy in American society, which prizes youth and health above all other values. The one million Americans who suffer the compound burdens of illness and advanced age are neglected and relegated to the bottom of the American social structure. But there is yet another group in the U.S. which is regarded as even less important and less valuable. If it is hell in America to be old and ill, it is something worse to be old and ill and black (or Asian, Indian, or Mexican).

There are thousands of blacks, Asian Americans, Indians, and Mexican Americans who face this triple jeopardy. Although they undoubtedly have need for the medical and nursing services provided in America's nursing homes, few of them are ever admitted to long term care facilities. In fact, while they make up almost 20 percent of the population, minorities account for only about four percent of the patients in America's nursing homes.

The Subcommittee on Long Term Care held hearings to determine why so few members of minority groups are admitted. Witnesses representing all minorities were asked to research the subject and present their views. There was a prompt consensus that four factors were involved: discrimination, cost, personal choice, and social and cultural differences. The relative importance of each of these factors varied greatly from group to group.

ELDERLY ASIANS

Elderly Asians are a diverse group made up of Japanese, Chinese, Filipinos, and Koreans. They number 1.5 million in the United States, about one million of whom live on the West Coast. They are bound together by their common problems and their common experiences in

117

this country. Most migrated to America at the turn of the century; most worked at hard labor. They suffered from racial discrimination and legal, social, and cultural barriers to assimilation.

Among these barriers were the Asian exclusion laws and the Gentlemen's Agreement of 1908, which prevented many of them from bringing their loved ones into this country. Other affronts included the internment of thousands of Japanese in detention camps in the early 1940s. Their answer to a society that made it clear they weren't wanted was a self-imposed isolation. This alienation assured the retention of the languages and customs of their native land.[1]

Another natural reaction to their rejection from the society of majority whites was a growing reputation for self-sufficiency. Even present-day Asian Americans who live in isolated pockets in our major cities are credited with "taking care of their own." This is required by the rich family tradition which commands veneration of the elderly.

Unfortunately, this reputation for self-reliance has been translated and perpetuated in the present-day mythology that the Asian Americans really have no problems. This is regrettable, because years of rejection, discrimination, and desolation undoubtedly have left many Asians hungering for assistance in their old age.

While there is clear need for nursing home care among elderly Asians, few receive it. The tradition which required that the elderly be respected has been eroded somewhat, but is still strong enough to require care for most in their homes. But since many Chinese were prevented by Asian exclusion laws from bringing their families into this country, there are substantial numbers who now have no one to take care of them. Despite the fact that some 20 percent of San Francisco's Chinatown are over 65, there is only one Chinese-owned and operated nursing home in that city.

Those unfortunate enough to fall into the hands of the state live to regret it. In the Bay Area, it means being shipped 50 or 60 miles out of the city to white-owned nursing homes in surrounding counties. Nursing home beds for Medicaid patients are notoriously scarce in San Francisco. Life for an elderly Asian in a nursing home run by whites can be a harrowing experience. Many find themselves among strangers unable to understand or to make themselves understood. This inability to communicate leads to increased neglect. The food is seldom, if ever, familiar or appetizing, and the customs are different. Too often, the result is tragedy. For example, the subcommittee received the following reports.

In one nursing home, an elderly Japanese woman was strapped to a wheelchair, presumably for her own protection. She was unable to speak any English, and there were no bilingual staff members. She was ignored most of the time. One day she was found dead from suffocation because the straps were too tight.

Another tragic incident involved an elderly Chinese woman in her 80s who refused to eat meals because the food was unfamiliar to her. She found the meals unappetizing. Unable to speak English, she could not explain why she could not eat her meals. The staff considered her behavior obstinate. This continued for several weeks until she had to be put in intensive care for malnutrition.

It is little wonder, then, that elderly Asians ranked language, social, and cultural factors as the most important reasons for their absence from nursing homes. Personal choice was ranked a strong second. San Francisco's respected Sam Yuen testified:

> Elderly Asian-Americans often associate going to these traditional nursing homes with going away to die because these homes make little or no effort to overcome the language and cultural barriers or truly rehabilitate them for return to their own homes and community. Once brought there, they are completely forgotten. The elderly have seen too many of their friends go away and never return. Nursing homes, therefore, have to them become "death houses" or "collection stations for the mortuary."

Asians testified that cost was not much of an obstacle since most of them could qualify for assistance through the Medicaid program. Discrimination was ranked as the fourth and last factor explaining Asian absence from nursing homes. It was pointed out, however, that no real confrontation had been made. Not many Asians have attempted to enter white-run nursing homes; thus, it is impossible to judge how many would be accepted or refused.

AGED BLACKS

Blacks in the U.S. make up about 10 percent of the population; about 1,750,000 of them are over 65. In the words of Compton, California's Dr. Hubert Hemsley, "their health indices reflect a lifetime of substandard housing, poverty, limited educational opportunities, lack of adequate medical and social resources which are the natural legacy of a society in which white supremacy and social Darwinism have been the philosophical basis for pathological decisions concerning blacks."[2]

Older blacks are twice as likely to be poor; 50 percent live in poverty as compared with 23 percent for whites. While over half of them continue to live in the South, the migration of this minority group into urban areas has created overcrowded conditions, poor sanitation, unemployment, maladjustment, poor health, drug addiction, and social and personal violence. To the black American this means a higher mortality rate at every stage of life. From 45 to 64, black women have twice the mortality rate of white women; from 55 to 64, the mortality for black men is ten percent higher than for white men. Despite higher incidences of acute and chronic disease, an elderly black sees a physician at an average annual rate of 4.9 visits as compared with a white's 6.1 visits. Dr. Hemsley comments that aged blacks are experiencing no temporary aberration, but rather the continuing effect of poverty and racism. "Now in their golden years, they have relinquished whatever hopes they had — resigned to an ignominious death in a subtle form of euthanasia."

The 1960 report of the Subcommittee on Problems of the Aged and Aging of the Senate Committee on Labor and Public Welfare took note of these problems and the particular absence of blacks from nursing homes. The report stressed that social and economic factors explained this absence and urged that the problem be given special attention. The problem has been given anything but special attention. Examples of discrimination against blacks appear throughout the hearings held by the Subcommittee on Long Term Care from 1963 to the present.

Dr. Hemsley stated his belief that discrimination was the most important factor explaining blacks' absence from nursing homes:

> I will have to agree with the Kerner Commission that the chief problem in this country is racism and it reflects itself in many areas. Why aren't there proportionate numbers of Blacks and minority people in nursing homes? The question is answered when you find out there aren't any nursing homes which they can own and operate with their life style. If the banking institutions, government enforcement agencies could give them the type of help they give the oil industry, Lockheed or Amtrack, if we could give this kind of "welfare" to the poor people, the problem would be solved, but what we have in this country is "welfare" for the rich and free enterprise for the poor.

Since half of the 1.7 million elderly blacks are poor, it appeared safe to assume that cost would *not* be an important factor, the assumption being that the poor are eligible for Medicaid, which now pays more than 50 percent of the nation's nursing home bill. Dr. Hobart Jackson, of the National Caucus of the Black Aged, quickly dispelled the notion. He said cost was the most important obstacle to nursing home care for blacks, although he gave discrimination almost equal status. He noted that many blacks did not understand that there was such a program as Medicaid or how to sign up for it. He noted that co-insurance and increasing out-of-pocket costs constitute a significant disincentive to use of the Medicare program. He added that comparatively few blacks were receiving Social Security because of their previous employment in agriculture or domestic services. "The new programs developed for the aging are no substitute for money, their greatest need," he said, noting in particular the absence of black owned and operated facilities.

While there are obvious social and cultural differences between blacks and the white majority population, these differences rank well behind cost and discrimination as a reason for blacks' not entering nursing homes. Like Asians, they continue to have a reputation for "taking care of their own." Representatives of the black community noted that this tradition continues for the principal reason that there is no place beyond the bosom of the family that an elderly black can find supportive services.

Blacks share a negative view of nursing homes according to witnesses before the subcommittee. But even so, personal choice ranks fourth and last as a reason that there are not more blacks in nursing homes. Dr. Jacquelyne Jackson testified, "Many Blacks have actually witnessed old Blacks dying in deplorable circumstances in various facilities through the years and a number believe that one would increase the possibility of dying in a degree of dignity and such death may best come by remaining at home."

ELDERLY INDIANS

There are about 500,000 Indians and Alaskan natives living on reservations in the U.S. Few Americans realize the stark deprivation of most Indians who have been pushed by whites onto what was considered the most worthless land in the United States. The Navajo reservation is typical. It occupies 25,000 square miles in the northeastern corner of Arizona, the northwestern corner of New Mexico, and the southeastern tip of Utah. The reservation is roughly the size of West Virginia, but much of the land is rough, desolate, and so rocky that it is of little economic benefit. While West Virginia has 26,000 miles of paved roads, the Navajo reservation has only 1,500, the rest are dirt roads, which are impassible when it rains or snows. While the reservation accommodates slightly less than one-third of the Indians in the U.S., they have a per capita income of $500 a year and an unemployment rate of 65 percent a year.

It is a picture of isolation and poverty. Medical necessities are scarce. As Roger Sandoval put it, "the nearest store is 40 miles away, but few Indians have automobiles; thus, help in an emergency is not just the turn of a key away." All too often, Indians who have died have not been found until five or six days later. Diseases which could have been arrested continue going untreated, taking their toll of human life and spreading misery.

Despite a great need, witnesses before the subcommittee knew of only three nursing homes on Indian reservations. The first is located at Pine Ridge, South Dakota, another on the Navajo reservation and a third, operated by a church, on the Gila River Reservation near Phoenix, Arizona. In fact, less than 200 nursing home beds are located on reservations, and if the need is conservatively established at one percent of the Indian population, there is a present shortage of 5,000 nursing home beds. To be sure, there are a few Indians in nursing homes located outside the reservation, but this alienation from friends, family, and familiar surroundings has not been attractive to the Indian. Given the choice between deprivation and need in familiar surroundings, or nursing services in unfamiliar surroundings, Indians choose the former.

Perry Swisher, director of Special Educational Services, Idaho State University at Pocatello, Idaho, wrote to the subcommittee:

> My extensive experience with elderly Indians has led me to the conclusion that the design and operation of rest homes are hostile to the Indian life style: The isolation from the rest of the community; separation from the young; the inconvenience of visits by a group of relatives; the food; the enforced uselessness; the sanitary preoccupations that eliminate any contact with livestock, wildlife, running water or ponds and open country in general.

The above quotation emphasizes why elderly Indians listed social and cultural differences as the number one reason for their absence from nursing homes. But there is yet another reason—Indians enjoy the services of medicine men. Roger Sandoval, of the Navajo Tribe, told the subcommittee, "Basically it is a type of care which relates to a great extent to the use of herbs and a little witchcraft maybe and they are quite successful and well respected citizens." The fact that some nursing homes have forbidden medicine men to visit the infirm is very unsettling to the Indians.

On the question of whether the Indians continue to venerate their elderly and provide care, witnesses were unanimous that the close family ties continue, and that care for the aged is provided by immediate family members. "It is not as close as it used to be a number of years ago because the younger generation is drifting into urban areas and getting away from their older folks, but it is still true to a great extent," said Mr. Sandoval.

The second most important reason that Indians do not seek nursing home care in greater numbers is that they cannot afford it. The problem is peculiar. Indian reservations are federal enclaves; this means that they are under the jurisdiction of the federal government. Accordingly, state governments have uniformly refused to license and inspect nursing homes on Indian reservations. Since state licensure of such facilities is a precondition to qualifying for Medicare or Medicaid funds, no Indians were receiving care under either of these two programs.

As the result of the Senate hearings, Senator Moss added an amendment to a pending Medicaid reform bill which requires the secretary of HEW to certify nursing homes on Indian reservations. The only problem now is that Indians still cannot find the money to construct the nursing homes on reservations as they would like to.

Personal choice ranks almost coequally with the other two reasons that more Indians are not in nursing homes. Dorothy G. Baker of Blackfoot, Idaho wrote to the subcommittee: "When an Indian is placed in a convalescent center, he is isolated, he goes into a state of mourning... they feel they are sent away to die."

Discrimination was ranked last by Indians, but like the Asians, they emphasized that not many Indians have tried to enter white-owned nursing homes. Thus, the question of possible discrimination remains open.

OLDER MEXICAN AMERICANS

There are approximately 12 million Mexican Americans in the United States. There are known to be over one million age 65 and over in two states alone—New Mexico and Texas. When Mexican Americans reach their golden years, they have already endured many hardships, including poverty, desolation, unemployment, and lack of adequate housing and health facilities.

Many older Mexican Americans have no electric lights, no running water, and inadequate toilet facilities. They suffer from high indices of arthritis and heart disease. Many still employ salt water and herbs to cure toothaches because they don't have the money to pay for dental care. Few can obtain the services of a nursing home, despite the obvious need.

Discrimination was ranked as the most important reason that greater numbers of older Mexican Americans are not in nursing homes. Corrine Garcia of Rocky Ford, Colorado, told the subcommittee:

> Nursing homes can, and do, discriminate against our people. In my hometown alone, 43 percent of the population are Mexican-Americans, 57 percent are Anglo. The Spanish percentage of the elderly is 13 percent. Yet in the nursing home there are only two Spanish-surnamed persons in the entire facility and it has 85 beds.

She told of calling nursing homes near her home and being told of vacancies. But upon giving the patient's name, Trujillio, the vacancies evaporated. After the repeated necessity of sending the elderly as far as 83 miles away from home, a discrimination suit against the Colorado Welfare Department made it possible to place Mexican American patients in her home town nursing home.

Cost was ranked second in importance by the experts before the subcommittee. Asked about the availability of the Medicaid program, Mexican American representatives told the senators that Medicaid is a well-kept secret among the Anglos (whites); it is administered by the Anglos for the Anglos. The language barrier and the lack of publications in Spanish were cited as significant deterrents to use of the Medicaid program.

Social and cultural differences also play an important role. Like the elders of other minority groups, Mexican American seniors, "viejitos," have been slow to aculturate and slow to learn English. If admitted to a nursing home, they find themselves surrounded by the Anglos who have taken advantage of them and exploited them for so many years. They are unable to communicate, and they find the food distasteful. But, if they will accept them at all, very few nursing homes make any separate provisions for them. The tradition of taking care of the elderly has been weakened somewhat with increased "Americanization," but is still the norm in the Mexican American community.

For those Mexican Americans who are admitted to a nursing home, it is not always the happiest of experiences. Anna Plasencia of Nampa, Idaho, wrote to the subcommittee, "A severe diabetic Mexican American lady with mental problems was admitted to a nursing home. It was a full year before the nursing home realized she was Mexican; they thought she was Indian. She was not able to communicate with anyone for the whole year." Consequently, if given the choice, most Mexican Americans will avoid nursing homes. Asked how nursing homes were viewed in her community, Sister Ramirez said, "They are viewed like jails."

ENFORCEMENT OF THE CIVIL RIGHTS ACT

Title VI of the Civil Rights Act of 1964 prohibits discrimination based on race, color, or national origin in any institution which receives federal assistance or participates in federally assisted programs. Nursing homes can receive federal financial assistance from some 50 programs and clearly fall within the purview of the act.

The primary responsibility for implementing Title VI lies with the Office of Civil Rights, part of the Office of the Secretary of HEW. After the office investigates, complaints which cannot be resolved are referred to the Civil Rights Division of the Department of Justice. The subcommittee's examination of the record revealed anything but an aggressive enforcement policy. The Office of Civil Rights reported that 710 nursing homes were surveyed between 1971 and 1972, with most homes found in compliance. It is not clear from the report whether the surveys were on-sight or paper examinations. There were 19 complaints which were investigated and resolved.[3]

Through 1972, the office of Civil Rights had not referred one case to the Department of Justice for prosecution. In fact, the only case that was brought by this agency against a nursing home was brought under Title VII, the fair housing section of the Civil Rights Act.

On September 17 and 24, 1973, Congressman Don Edwards, chairman of the House Committee on the Judiciary's Subcommittee on Civil and Constitutional Rights, conducted hearings reaching the same conclusion: "Too long Blacks, Spanish Americans and other members of racial and ethnic groups have been denied equal access to hospitals and nursing homes." On September 16, the GAO presented to that subcommittee its report confirming Mr. Edward's conclusion and showing that a dual system of health care still exists for nonwhites despite the enactment of Title VI of the Civil Rights Act. Significantly, as of

December 1976, HEW's Office of Civil Rights still had not referred to the Department of Justice one case against a nursing home for prosecution under Title VI, the applicable section of the Civil Rights Act.

Conclusion

There is a demonstrated need for nursing home care among the minorities of this country, but little help has been forthcoming. In spite of the fact that many minority aged are poor, they have not had the same access to the Medicaid program as whites. Accordingly, inability to pay is an important factor in explaining their absence from nursing homes. Differing social customs and language play an important role, as does personal choice. But perhaps most important in explaining the absence of minorities from nursing homes is discrimination. It is a sad commentary that Title VI of the Civil Rights Act of 1964, which prohibits such discrimination, has not been enforced by either HEW or the Department of Justice.

The provisions of the Civil Rights Act must be enforced. Nursing homes should make a greater effort to gain the confidence of minority groups by accepting social and cultural differences and honoring their traditions. Anything less will constitute a ratification of the existing policy of deprivation and discrimination toward those who now face the triple jeopardies of age, illness, and racial discrimination en route to an ignominious death.

Chapter 8

How Many Nursing Homes Are Substandard?

The next obvious question is: How many nursing homes have such problems? How many are substandard; that is, how many have serious and life-threatening (as opposed to technical) violations?

After studying the question for more than seven years, holding some 25 hearings, and compiling 3,000 pages of testimony, the Subcommittee on Long Term Care concluded on the weight of the evidence that over 50 percent of the nursing homes in the United States are substandard. This judgment, first offered in December 1974 after a poll of the subcommittee membership, remains valid today.

Given the operation of the present system, it could hardly be otherwise. As will be seen in forthcoming chapters, the United States has no clear and consistent policy for treating the infirm elderly. State Medicaid reimbursement formulas contain financial incentives that encourage poor care. Physicians avoid nursing homes; nurses are few and far between. Thus, 80 to 90 percent of the care is being given by untrained and unlicensed aides and orderlies. Finally, the inspection and enforcement system is not working; among other liabilities, it is greatly hampered by political interference.

The inescapable result is poor care and abuse, of which the preceding chapters are merely illustrative. Thousands of similar examples are contained in the subcommittee's files. These files are the first source of support for the judgment that 50 percent of U.S. nursing homes are substandard. The files contain information obtained from many diverse sources, such as state health departments, patients or families, physicians, vendors, visitors, and nursing home owners. The bulk of the data is complaints sent to congressional committees and to individual members of Congress. Many of these complaints were addressed to the subcommittee; literally thousands of others were referred by other congressional offices. Upon investigation of these complaints, the subcommittee staff found most of them to be valid. The experience of HEW's ombudsman program, funded initially in five states, adds credibility. Program directors investigated 1,196 complaints about nursing homes in one year and found 80 percent of them to be justified.

A second source of support is the more than 60 major newspaper exposés on nursing homes in the past ten years. The similarity of charges in hard-hitting investigations by the *New York Times*, the *Chicago Tribune*, the *Milwaukee Journal*, and the *St Petersburg* (Florida) *Times*, is notable. More often than not, the findings of the press have been confirmed by follow-up investigations conducted by state or federal agencies.

A third source of support is the judgments and conclusions of experts. For example, Dr. J. Raymond Gladue, president of the American Association of Nursing Home Physicians, testified in October 1973 that the quality of care in U.S. nursing homes was "either very poor or scandalous." He added that he had seen little improvement in the past five years. In his 1973 appearance before the subcommittee, Nelson Cruikshank, president of the National Council of Senior Citizens, described conditions in the nation's nursing homes as "nothing short of a national scandal." In 1971, the executive council of the AFL-CIO issued a statement protesting the "heartless indifference, cruelty, neglect and financial exploitation in U.S. nursing homes." Bert Seidman, speaking for the AFL-CIO, charged that four out of five (80 percent) nursing homes are in violation of federal and state standards. In February 1976, the union adopted another resolution, protesting the continuing crisis in nursing home care and calling for a national investigation of nursing homes. In March 1977, they issued a scathing report calling for a crackdown and recommending that federal funds be limited to nonprofit nursing homes.

Independent studies provide a fourth source of support. Among the most important of these was the Nader task force report issued in 1970 which charged that "80 percent of the nursing homes receiving Federal tax dollars were substandard."

Governor David Pryor of Arkansas (a former congressman) concluded on the basis of his own study that 80 percent of U.S. nursing homes had serious violations. During the subcommittee's November 1971 hearings in Minnesota (a leading state in terms of health care delivery), Daphne Krause, executive director of the Minneapolis Age and Opportunity Center, concluded that 40 of the 125 (about 30 percent) homes evaluated during her six-year investigation had serious violations. Other similar reports (e.g., the 1975 Connecticut report) have been produced by various public interest research groups.

A fifth source of support is studies conducted by state governments. In 1971, the Better Government Association, which worked with the staff of the subcommittee in evaluating Illinois nursing homes and state inspection records, concluded that 50 percent of the state's homes had serious, life-threatening deficiencies. Chicago officials admitted that 45 percent of its homes were substandard. The Cook County Department of Public Welfare verified the BGA's charge concerning 100 homes in its jurisdiction. The Illinois Department of Health concurred in the BGA charge. Similarly, the lieutenant governor of Wisconsin, in his 1971 report, charged that 51 of Milwaukee's 99 nursing homes had serious violations; 35 homes had violations so serious to merit their immediate closing. In Florida, State Senator Louis de La Parte, chairman of the joint ad hoc committee to investigate nursing homes, disclosed that "40 out of the almost 100 nursing homes investigated did not meet basic requirements."

In November of 1975, the attorney general of Kansas presented to the subcommittee a report documenting significant abuses in his state. Speaking of the subcommittee's report charging that 50 percent of U.S. nursing homes are substandard, the attorney general stated, "It should be noted that this study established, time and time again, that those findings of the Subcommittee on Long-Term Care of the U.S. Senate Special Committee on Aging were not foreign to the State of Kansas."

In June of 1975, Max Factor, hearing examiner in the office of Los Angeles city attorney, Burt Pines, issued his report:

> Patient care conditions at Los Angeles nursing homes are often inadequate and shocking. [Our] hearings were replete with graphic examples of patient mistreatment and abuse, inadequate diet, and poor food preparation, misuse of medications, the theft of patient property and reprisals against patients who complain.

Additional reports were issued in January 1976 by the joint House-Senate Committee on Nuring Homes of the Minnesota Legislature and in October 1976 by New Jersey's Special Commission on Investigations.

Similarly, in New York, a 1973 study by the state health department revealed that nearly two-thirds of New York City's 104 nursing homes had serious operating deficiencies. These findings were confirmed by the subcommittee's 1975 hearings in New York. Added support was supplied by the seven-volume report of the New York State Moreland Act Commission on Nursing Homes and Residential Facilities. Finally, in his November 1976 testimony before the subcommittee, Charles J.

Hynes, New York's special prosecutor, testified that 50 percent of the city's nursing homes may be receiving kickbacks from local vendors.

Studies by independent agencies are a sixth source of support. For example, in 1971, the GAO concluded that over 50 percent of the nursing homes surveyed in three states—Oklahoma, New York, and Michigan—did not meet minimum standards of fire safety, nursing care, and physicians' services. In November 1972, another GAO report stated, "The quality of care in U.S. nursing homes is still far too low." on June 11, 1974, the GAO presented testimony before a subcommittee of the House Government Operations Committee relating to its eleven-state investigation of nursing home fire safety. The GAO reported that 72 percent of the sampled nursing homes had one or more major fire safety deficiencies. On August 31, 1976, Senator Moss released the results of yet another GAO audit relating to the handling of patients' funds by nursing homes in five states. *Every home in GAO's sample* had significant problems with protecting the integrity of patients' funds. The question of the handling of patients' funds is only one in a series of issues to be examined in a full-scale examination of the nursing home industry announced in September of 1976 by the Federal Trade Commission. According to the present chairman, Mike Pertschuk, the nonpublic investigation will take two years to complete.

A seventh support is the findings and pronouncements from the executive branch, specifically HEW and the White House. In a June 1971 speech, President Nixon noted that "many U.S. nursing homes are little more than warehouses for the dying." The president's words were amplified by Undersecretary John Veneman, who appeared before the subcommittee in October 1971. When asked how many nursing homes are substandard, with life-threatening conditions, he responded:

> The question is difficult to respond to. The sample taken by the GAO indicated roughly a 50 percent figure in the Medicaid institutions they investigated were not complying with standards established by the program. As I pointed out in my testimony, it will vary from state to state. You will find some states where the ratio will be higher.

Art Hess, deputy director of the Social Security Administration, testified in the same hearing that of the 4,339 nursing homes participating in Medicare, only 1,141 had no serious violations. In short, 73 percent had serious violations. The data he supplied indicated that the violations were protracted. During the period of September 1968 through December 1971, at least 70 percent of the participating homes continuously had major deficiencies.

In January of 1974, Dr. Faye G. Abdellah, director of the Office of Nursing Home Affairs, announced that 59 percent of the nation's 7,000 skilled nursing homes did not meet federal minimum fire safety standards. Dr. Abdellah charged that an even higher percentage of the nation's 8,000 intermediate care facilities do not meet the fire standards. In April of 1975, HEW announced a detailed audit of nursing homes. The report notes that two-thirds of the nursing homes surveyed had several (more than four) fire safety deficiencies. (In December 1976 HEW claimed 47 percent deficiencies.)

Clearly, the Subcommittee on Long Term Care had compelling evidence to support its conclusion that 50 percent of the nursing homes in the United States are substandard. Indeed, the conclusion would be supportable if the only data available were the GAO and HEW studies showing that 72 and 66 percent (respectively) of American nursing homes were deficient just from the point of view of fire safety.

Obviously, there is some variation from state to state in the quality of care. But in the final analysis, the precise percentage of substandard homes is not the issue. If only a fringe of the nation's 23,000 long term care facilities were substandard, there would still be a desperate need for reform. The time for denials and mutual recriminations is long past. It is time for operators and consumer advocates to work together in the spirit of trust and good will if there is ever to be any improvement in the quality of life for our one million elderly and ill Americans.

But a basic understanding of the problem is essential to reform. Having discovered *what* happens in nursing homes, it is now time to learn *why* it happens.

Part II
Root Causes of Nursing Home Abuses

Part I of this book is a description of what happens in America's 23,000 nursing homes. Part II is an explanation of why it happens. America has yet to decide what to do with its ailing aged. The rhetoric is of care and concern, but the reality is indecision, confusion, and ineffective, piecemeal programs. It is clear that the inspection and enforcement machinery is not working and that one substantial obstruction is political interference. Moreover, the present system of reimbursing nursing home operators provides built-in financial incentives which guarantee poor care. Finally, it is just as apparent that physicians have abdicated their responsibility for nursing home patients and that nurses are scarce; consequently, untrained and unlicensed aides and orderlies provide 80 to 90 percent of the care.

Chapter 9
Lack of Policy Toward the Infirm Elderly

If there is unanimous agreement anywhere in the field of long term care, it is that the United States lacks any kind of comprehensive and consistent policy with respect to the infirm elderly. The phenomenon of large numbers of ill aged is a fairly recent development in America, and we have never really come to grips with it.

The need for a comprehensive policy was recognized as far back as 1959 when the Senate Subcommittee on the Problems of the Aging and Aged issued its landmark report. Two years later, the White House Conference on Aging resolved that there was a need which should be met by making the broad spectrum of institutional and in-home services available to the elderly.

Since that time, there have been some gains, principally through the enactment of the Medicare and Medicaid programs in 1965, but the benefits provided are still woefully short of what is needed. These conclusions were underscored in 1970 by the blue ribbon Task Force on Medicaid and Related Problems, which commented:

> Long-Term care is a neglected and underdeveloped area. Medicare and Medicaid are not effective and efficient mechanisms for dealing with the problems...[T]he failure to address the problem directly distorts the operation and inflates the costs of the medical care programs.

The shortcomings of existing programs can also be indicated through statistics. According to the best estimates, over one-fifth of our 21 million older Americans require some degree of protective services, ranging from personal care (such as help in dressing, bathing, and eating) to intensive nursing intervention known as skilled nursing care. Of the some 4½ million older Americans who need help, only about 1½ million receive it. Most who do find assistance are in nursing homes. The remaining 3 million older Americans who are housebound, bedfast, or get around with difficulty are going without the care they need.

To be more precise, some 600,000 seniors need nursing home care which they cannot afford, while another 2.4 million need in-home services. Both home health care and nursing home care are authorized under Medicare and Medicaid, however, except for nursing home care under Medicaid, the level of funding has been very low. Outlay for home health is miniscule, accounting for about one percent of either program.

MEDICARE

Congress authorized nursing home care to all older Americans under Medicare as a less expensive alternative to keeping patients in hospitals during their convalescence. As implemented during the Johnson administration, individuals had to be hospitalized for at least three days in a row, a physician had to certify that they were eligible for and required "skilled nursing care," and they had to be admitted to a Medicare participating facility within 14 days of their discharge from the hospital. Stimulated by rising costs in this program, the Nixon administration in 1969 sought to cut back benefits. By administrative regulation they added two more requirements which prospective beneficiaries had to meet. First, they were required to have "rehabilitative potential," which was a euphemism for eliminating all terminal patients. Second, the words "skilled nursing care" were defined in narrow insurance terms to include only a very limited number of diagnoses and therapeutic situations. The effect of these regulations was virtually to make nursing home care unavailable to the elderly even though the Medicare literature continued to carry the promise of Congress that seniors were entitled to 120 days care in a nursing home.

Medicare's payments to nursing homes will total about $275 million in 1976, or something like two percent of all nursing home revenues. Only about 8,300 of the over one million patients in nursing homes on any given day will have their care paid for by Medicare. Expenditures for home health care in Medicare came to about $245 million, which was about one and a half percent of the $17.8 billion spent for Medicare in 1976.

MEDICAID

Medicaid is a much criticized grant-in-aid program administered by HEW in which the government pays from 50 to 78 percent of the cost incurred by the states in providing health care to those unable to pay for it. The largest share (38 percent) goes to pay for nursing home care. The elderly qualify only if they are essentially without income or assets.

In 1975, nursing homes received over $5 billion from Medicaid's $15 billion total. As the result of a 1967 amendment offered by Senator Moss, Medicaid authorizes payment for home health services. But funding has never reached even one percent of the total program.

The failure to fund home health programs is truly tragic, because these programs can serve to help maintain seniors in independence in their own homes where they most want to be; they can help prevent or postpone institutionalization. In addition, in-home services are generally a cheaper intervention than nursing home care. This fact has been aptly demonstrated by Daphne Krause, executive director of the successful Minneapolis Age and Opportunity Center (M.A.O.). She provides the following case history contrasting in-home services with nursing home placement:

Supportive Services for Mrs. M.R. over 3 years by M.A.O:
    Meals, including delivery charges
        (2 meals a day, 7 days a week) $3,385.00
    Housekeeping services (3 services a month)   399.60
    Counseling (average once a month)............324.00
      Total cost of M.A.O. services $4,008.00

Nursing Home costs for 3-year period
(projected cost):
$450.00 per month for 3 years...............$16,200.00
Less client's income of $115/month for 3
    years (client would be allowed to keep
    $25.00 a month for personal needs) ....-4,140.00
Remaining cost to be paid by Medicaid 12,060.00
Less cost of M.A.O. services ....-4,008.60
    Total M.A.O. saved the taxpayers over
    3 years with respect to a patient
    ordered institutionalized 8,051.40

Pronouncements about the value of home health services continue to be uttered by policy makers at all levels. For example, President Nixon told the 1971 White House Conference on Aging, "The greatest need is to help more older Americans go on living in their own homes." But this presidential promise was never fulfilled. It is symptomatic of our lack of a coherent policy that reality never follows rhetoric, and older Americans continue to suffer without the services they need.

Other indications of this failure can be seen in the absence of adult day care or holiday admittance programs, which are available in other nations. Many families would gladly keep their loved ones at home if they could afford to do so. Day care or a program to subsidize home care for needy elderly may be desirable options not now available. It is paradoxical that as a nation, we are willing to pay as much as $15,000 a year to keep a patient in a New York nursing home but are unwilling to pay the family $1,000 a year to help provide for their loved one at home. At the very least, we might consider allowing families who keep their elderly at home a tax deduction on home health expenses, even if the elderly do not qualify as dependents.

Besides overreliance on institutionalization, there are a great many other manifestations of our failure to establish a comprehensive policy toward the elderly. As a nation, we seem to be caught between two objectives, caring for the aged and protecting the property rights of businessmen. Courts and state health departments are reluctant to close down a home even in the face of serious and protracted violations. The rationale that is given is that closing a home would put the operator out of business; it would deprive him of his property and his livelihood. The frequency with which state agencies come down on the side of the entrepreneur and ignore the dire circumstances of patients is a reflection of the currently confused, inconsistent, and bankrupt policy we have toward the infirm elderly.

There are others who contend that the fact that we allow 80 percent of our nursing homes to operate for profit is the supreme example of our failure to come to grips with a policy which emphasizes people over profit. Critics charge that there is a fundamental contradiction between the goals of our society and the goals of for-profit nursing homes. It is said that the goal of society must be to rehabilitate patients and to return them to the community, while profitmaking nursing homes, if they prosper, must keep their beds full. Thus homes will tend to retain people in their facilities. It is charged that in a for-profit facility, dollars are the primary goal; patient care is a by-product of the search for dollars and profits. By contrast, patient care is the entire reason for nonprofit facilities' being.[1]

These critics may be right. The extent to which patient needs are sacrificed to business needs is obvious. Second, there are proportionately more fine nonprofit than for-profit homes. Moreover, nonprofit homes, on the average, spend more money per patient per day for food and for nursing personnel. But some homes use nonprofit status as a guise to attract new customers by converting what would be high profits into high salaries and other amenities for corporate officers. A 1972 HEW study shows that nonprofit homes are genuinely nonprofit in that most run in the red, and emphasizes that nonprofit homes on the average have almost double the labor expenses reported by for-profit homes. They also spend a larger portion of their total expenses for labor than do for-profit homes (65 percent of total costs as compared with 55 percent of total costs in for-profit facilities). With more personnel, particularly more registered nurses, on the average, the quality of care cannot help but be higher in nonprofit homes.

Those who argue the other side of the question carry the banner of pragmatism. They note that 80 percent of American nursing homes now operate for profit and that it would be practically impossible either to start from scratch again on a new system or to convert the massive number of homes into philanthropic entities. Indeed, they argue that the profit motive may be necessary to make *any* services available to the infirm aged. They point out that the present proprietary system had its roots in the enactment of the Social Security Act of 1935 and the universal condemnation of public poor houses. But, they assert, it was not only the bad track record of public institutions which led to the growth of for-profit nursing homes, it was also the failure of philanthropy to step in and fill the vacuum. Even today there is no major emphasis on philanthropy to provide services for the chronically ill.

The assertion that the profit motive per se is inconsistent with good nursing care would be easily acceptable if there were no for-profit nursing homes which offered excellent care. But there are some excellent proprietary homes. However, one thing is certain. The structure of reimbursement systems in most states tends to distort the operation of the free enterprise system, providing U.S. nursing homes with direct built-in financial incentives in favor of poor care.

FINANCIAL INCENTIVES TO POOR CARE

The General Accounting Office has been sharply critical of the way that states have reimbursed nursing homes. The basic problem is that rates have been determined arbitrarily. Most states have accepted

what operators claimed were their costs with no real independent effort to learn what should be an adequate rate of payment. In 1972, Congress required the states to adopt cost-related reimbursement formulas for nursing homes participating in the Medicaid program.
Regulations were announced implementing this law on July 1, 1976,
but the states have until 1978 to put them into effect. As generally in-
terpreted, the states can still pay nursing homes in any of the following ways providing they can plausibly demonstrate to HEW that their
formulas are somehow based upon costs.

The Flat Fee System

Many states have given operators a flat fee of perhaps $18 a day per
patient and taken it for granted that operators would use appropriate
amounts of this money for food, nursing care, housekeeping, and the
like. The virtue of this approach is that it provides the states a way of
controlling costs and fixes precise limits on the level of state obligations to nursing homes in any one year. The disadvantage is that this
system encourages homes to cut back on essential services, because
what is not spent becomes profit. Dr. John Knowles, for many years
director of the Massachusetts General Hospital in Boston, comments
that flat fee systems "only serve to reward poor homes who are not
providing the necessary services and turn a handsome profit while
good homes which do provide the services are penalized."

Cost-Related Reimbursement

Many states repay operators for the reasonable costs they have expended, usually up to certain maximum amounts per patient per day.
In short, whatever the operator spends, plus a return on the investment, will be paid subject to a very few limitations. Under this system,
there is (1) no incentive to keep costs down, (2) no relationship between
the dollars paid and the quality of care received, and (3) no controls on
the amount of state money obligated from year to year.

In its 1973 brief before the U.S. District Court for the District of Columbia, the Cost of Living Council (established to keep inflation in
check) criticized this type of reimbursement formula which is universally used in the federal Medicare program. The council charged that
there is "an incentive to incur marginally worthwhile expenditures
and then to attempt to justify their reimbursement—which has been
all too forthcoming."

An HEW study released shortly thereafter caused still more worries by concluding that Medicare homes had higher revenue levels

with below average occupancy rates, whereas the opposite is the rule. The report said, in part:

> Cost reimbursement techniques may not only encourage generally inefficient operations, but may encourage the maintenance of higher prices (and costs) during periods when competitive forces would induce them to lower them. That is, if (Medicare nursing home) operators can secure higher prices simply by keeping operating costs at a high level, they will tend to do so without regard to market demand forces.

The Cost of Living Council further extended this point by comparing average Medicare and Medicaid rates paid to nursing homes.

The average U.S. Medicaid reimbursement in 1970 was $11.23 per day as compared to $26.82 under Medicare. In 1971, Medicaid paid $13.52; Medicare paid $30.13. And in 1972, Medicaid paid $14.42, while Medicare paid $32.70 a day. The council further noted that when Michigan and Massachusetts switched from a flat fee system to a cost-based reimbursement system, the cost of the program in both states jumped dramatically.

If further worries about cost-related reimbursement were needed, they were provided during January 1975 subcommittee hearings in New York. After reviewing the evidence, Senator Moss said the formula was so generous as to "make defense contractors drool with envy. Virtually every expense is reimbursable including legal fees charged to fight the State Health Department from imposing sanctions on the home." Another glaring weakness was the absence of field audits to investigate and verify charges presented to Medicaid. Predictably, investigations and audits in New York have revealed that operators charged Medicaid for the purchase of mink coats, hi-fi sets, theater and sports tickets, paintings by Matisse and Renoir, vacations to Europe and Hawaii, investments in stocks and mutual funds, yachts, and Mercedes. The charges had been presented as business-related "travel and entertainment" expenses or were camouflaged as "dues and subscriptions."

Prospective Reimbursement

Colorado has a type of payment plan in which rates for the coming year are determined on an individual home-by-home basis after reviewing the previous year's CPA-audited financial statements. Rates are based upon costs plus almost a dollar per patient per day profit for the operator. This formula provides more accountability than the preceding formula, but there is still no relationship between the dollars paid and the quality of care. Fiscal manipulations, such as incurring higher and higher amounts of reimbursable costs, take precedence over patient care.

The Connecticut Points System

In this system, the focus is on the ability of the home to meet or exceed federal and state standards. Homes are assigned a certain number of points if they comply with particular standards; points are deducted for violating regulations. Bonus points are offered for exceeding criteria. Nursing homes are then graded and put into categories based on total performance. Class A nursing homes receive about one dollar more per patient per day than a Class B facility. The Class B home would receive about one dollar per patient per day more than a Class C home, and so on down the line. Under this system, the better the nursing home, the higher the rate of reimbursement. The weakness of this formula is that it stresses the home's capability to provide good care; it does not attempt to grade homes on the basis of the quality of care that they provide.

The Illinois Points System

This approach focuses on the patient and assigns points for each item of the patient's disability. The greater the degree of disability, the more a nursing home is reimbursed. The concept is rooted in an attempt to persuade nursing home operators to accept and provide good care for so-called "heavy care" patients who require unusual amounts of attention and who, therefore, are very costly to the facility. In practice however, the Illinois formula provides the classic example of the existence of financial incentives to poor care. When a patient qualifies for skilled nursing care, the state pays a base figure of about $600 a month. For each item of disability thereafter, the nursing home is paid $6 a point.

Under this system, a bed sore is worth eight points. If the operator allows the patients to develop bedsores, he can count on receiving $48 a month in addition to the base of $600. Moreover, if a patient is not helped to go to the bathroom and becomes incontinent of bowel and bladder, such condition is worth six points, or $36 more a month. Continuous catheterization itself is worth another eight points, or $48 more a month.

If, upon being left in his own wastes, a patient becomes bellicose, he can be labeled a behavioral problem worth eight points, or $48. Behavioral problems are routinely treated with tranquilizer drugs such as Thorazine or Mellaril. The daily administration of drugs is worth three points, or $18. If the drug is administered through injections rather than by mouth, another four points, or $24, are added onto the cost to the state.

The patient reduced to inactivity by drugs may be worth another three points if he is "completely dependent on staff or his condition is such that more than one staff member is required to give assistance" — another $18. Finally, the patient who is totally dependent and needs to be fed constantly is worth another four points, or $24 more per month.

The possibilities for the abuse of this system by the unscrupulous operator are obvious. Adding all of these contingencies it is possible to boost the rate paid by the state in excess of $1,000 per patient per month. This system actually encourages poor care. The unscrupulous operator has a direct financial interest in seeing patients become more disabled.

Senator Percy pointed out the folly of using this type of a reimbursement formula in the context of our present for-profit system. He asked Dr. Bruce Flashner, deputy director of the Illinois Department of Public Health, "What incentive is there to get patients out of bed, when there is a $48 per month extra payment for patients with bed sores?" Dr. Flashner responded:

> I totally agree with you, and I will not defend the point system. I think from not only a philosophical but from a practical point of view, it is insane to approach the problem that way. The point system probably was developed like most things with good intentions.... Of course, at the time they did not realize, as you pointed out, there was an incentive to keep people in their bed.

Five years after this conversation took place, this formula is still in effect in Illinois.

The Lack of Accountability

It is obvious that none of the reimbursement formulas are tied directly to the quality of care that is offered. Connecticut is the only state which attempts to provide positive incentives, but the efforts are geared to compliance with standards, not actual care delivered. Only Colorado has any sort of financial accountability. Given the increasing commitment of federal and state dollars to nursing homes, this lack of

fiscal responsibility is truly alarming and has far-reaching consequences.

The January 1975 disclosures concerning the lack of audits in New
York resulted in dramatic changes. Today, auditors from the Office of
Special Prosecutor for Nursing Homes have identified $70 million in
overpayments to nursing homes. But a closer look indicated that 21
states had never audited a single nursing home provider from the
beginning of the Medicaid program in 1966 through January 1976.[2]
Table 9-1 provides a state-by-state tally.

Table 9-1 Number of Medicaid Facilities Audited by State
Organizations

State	#	State	#
Alabama	55	Montana	1
Alaska	0	Nebraska	0
Arizona	0	Nevada	16
Arkansas	0	New Hampshire	25
California	0	New Jersey	316
Colorado	1	New Mexico	36
Connecticut	0	New York	222
Delaware	24	North Carolina	87
District of Columbia	0	North Dakota	0
Florida	0	Ohio	4
Georgia	0	Oklahoma	0
Hawaii	NA	Oregon	57
Idaho	3	Pennsylvania	319
Illinois	398	Puerto Rico	0
Indiana	0	Rhode Island	27
Iowa	0	South Carolina	38
Kansas	36	South Dakota	0
Kentucky	94	Tennessee	60
Louisiana	206	Texas	375
Maine	75	Utah	0
Maryland	543	Vermont	0
Massachusetts	600	Virginia	170
Michigan	1370	Washington	0
Minnesota	51	West Virginia	0
Mississippi	0	Wisconsin	487
Missouri	350	Wyoming	0

WHAT MUST BE DONE

What is clearly needed is a reversal of the financial incentives so that good nursing home care is encouraged. The Connecticut system is a good start, but it should be broadened beyond rewarding the development of the capacity to provide good care. It is possible to determine reasonable therapeutic goals for every patient admitted to a nursing home. Nursing homes are already required to establish treatment plans for each patient. After a certain period of time, a medical review team composed of a physician, a social worker, and a nurse should evaluate how successful the home has been in reaching the therapeutic goals established for the patient.

Adding this measurement of the actual care delivered into the formula which measures the home's capacity to deliver good care, nursing homes would receive an aggregate grade and a ranking. The better the nursing home, the higher the levels of reimbursement. Under this approach, there would be direct financial incentives to good care. Dr. John Knowles and other experts have recommended this system because it rewards good homes and penalizes poor ones.

But this or any system of paying nursing homes must also offer public accountability. Nursing homes should be required to provide CPA-audited financial statements and to certify that the costs presented are accurate and appropriate for reimbursement from Medicaid. Penalties of $10,000 fine and a year in jail should be provided for false statements. The federal government must insist that states conduct field audits of all nursing homes at least once every two years.

These improvements must be only part of a concerted effort to establish a comprehensive and workable policy toward the infirm elderly. At the heart of such a policy should be expanded in-home services to keep seniors independent in their own homes until they actually require placement in long term care facilities. For those who need the intensive care offered by nursing homes, there should be appropriate federal assistance available.

Chapter 10
Enforcement of Standards: A National Farce

By the end of World War II, every state had enacted legislation creating standards for the operation of nursing homes, providing penalties for noncompliance and designating some state agency to oversee enforcement. Unfortunately, these systems, with few exceptions, have never been effective. It was true in 1960 when a report of the Senate Subcommittee on Problems of the Aged and Aging charged, "Licensure standards differ greatly and are either too low or not being enforced," and it is true today as evidenced by the fact that 50 percent of all U.S. nursing homes have serious violations. The principal reason this is true is that the Department of Health, Education, and Welfare has abdicated its responsibility under the law to set and enforce federal mininum standards, relying instead on the anemic enforcement of the states (at least through January 1977).

HEW'S DEFAULT ON STANDARDS AND ENFORCEMENT

The subcommittee's 1965 hearings documented that standards differed greatly among the states and that there was an even greater disparity in the manner and vigor of state enforcement. The conclusion that state enforcement was generally ineffective greatly reinforced the need for federal minimum standards and federal enforcement to follow the increasing flow of federal dollars into nursing homes. However, Medicaid was enacted without federal standards in that year, and while authority for uniform federal minimum standards were added to Medicare, enforcement was left in the hands of the states.

In 1967, several members of the Committee on Aging overcame the cry of federal intervention and were successful in adding both federal minimum standards and enforcement authority to the Medicaid program. These amendments to the 1967 Social Security Act were labeled the Moss and Kennedy amendments. The Moss provisions gave the secretary of HEW wide enforcement authority to ensure that federal funds did not go to substandard facilities. They required the disclosure of nursing home ownership and established minimum nurse staffing and comprehensive fire safety and dietary requirements. Senator Edward M. Kennedy's amendment required the licensure of nursing home administrators.

Unfortunately, as so often happens, the battles won on the floor of the Senate were lost in the *Federal Register.* In other words, Congress writes the law in broad strokes, leaving it to the administrative agency (HEW) to fill in the details and translate to the nursing home operators exactly what they have to do. In this case, HEW simply has not lived up to its responsibility. The law required operators to be in compliance with the new standards by January 1, 1969, but it was May 1970, a year and a half later, before HEW issued the first standards in implementation of the 1967 amendments.

During May 1970 hearings, Val Halamandaris charged HEW with "indifference if not outright culpable neglect" because of their 2½ year delay in the implementation of standards. He used the term "bureaucratic lawlessness" to describe HEW's failure to use the enforcement authority provided by the statute. HEW's failure to implement other important provisions, such as medical review (a patient-by-patient evaluation of the quality of care by a team of health professionals), was examined against evidence showing that HEW had assigned 122 people and expended 40 worker years to write federal standards for the Medicare nursing home program but less than two worker years to write standards for the much larger Medicaid program.

The inadequacy of nursing personnel standards and specifically, the absence of minimum patient-nurse ratios was discussed in the context of a disclosure that a consultant hired by HEW to help write the regulations was, at the same time, employed as a consultant to the American Nursing Home Association.

The subcommittee sought to clarify congressional intent with respect to the Kennedy amendment requiring the licensure of nursing home administrators. The law was enacted because of 1965 data showing inadequate state legislation in this field. In fact, 13 states did not mention the administrator in their regulations; another 10 referred to him only by title; 28 states had no educational, training, or experience requirements; and only 22 required that the administrator be of good moral character. The statute required states to establish licensure boards including representatives of professions and institutions concerned with the care of the chronically ill and aged. The legislative history was clear that the boards were not to be dominated by the nursing home industry or any other groups. Senator Stephen Young of Ohio put it best: "Licensure of nursing homes by operators is as good as regulation of saloons by bartenders." It was, therefore, inexplicable why HEW issued regulations allowing nursing home operators to make up a majority of the licensure boards.

For their part, HEW witnesses apologized for the delay but, other than referring to forthcoming preliminary standards for medical review, refused to give any assurances as to when or if subsequent standards would be issued. Apparently, they took little note of the subcommittee's insistence that the secretary of HEW was in default of his responsibility under the 1967 amendments to ensure that federal funds did not go to substandard facilities. Apparently, they also took little note of the subcommittee's concern that administrators were dominating state licensure boards. Subsequent HEW data given to William R. Hutton, executive director of the National Council of Senior Citizens, disclosed that operators were in the majority on the boards of 21 states and were, with the assistance of members who might have an interest in nursing homes, in a position to dominate the boards of 40 states.

In December of 1970, Ralph Nader and his task force testified before the subcommittee and, having reviewed HEW's handling of the enforcement of the Moss and Kennedy amendments of 1967, asked the subcommittee "to consider personal sanctions to individuals who have, in effect, so seriously neglected their jobs or so willfully neglected enforcing the law that their very tenure in office must be brought into question."

In 1971, more and more consumer and senior citizen spokesmen were critical of HEW's enforcement of the law. Several studies were produced showing that 50 to 80 percent of U.S. nursing homes did not meet minimum standards, including the now-famous May 1971 General Accounting Office audit of New York, Michigan, and Oklahoma. In addition, the subcommittee itself accumulated increasing evidence to support the premise that perhaps 50 percent of the nursing homes in the U.S. were substandard. Moreover, these studies showing high incidences of substandard facilities also indicated that few homes were closed, further evidence of the overall failure of the enforcement system. In Illinois, for example, where 50 percent of the nursing homes were found to be substandard, three homes were closed between 1961 and 1971; in New York, 20 administrative hearings were held and two homes closed; in Maryland, no homes were closed through the formal legal proceedings, and only three homes were closed in Minnesota from 1954 through 1971.

In June 1971, the weight of these facts came to the attention of President Nixon, who promised to eliminate substandard nursing homes and turn them into "shining symbols of hope." To carry out his "gameplan" he turned to HEW, the agency perhaps most to blame for the existing problems. The obvious questions from the point of view of patient advocates were: Is the president serious? and Can HEW handle the job? The following excerpt from a confidential memo from then Secretary of HEW Elliot Richardson to the president proves that HEW was aware of its responsibility and default under the 1967 Moss and Kennedy amendments:

> Since about 40 percent of the funds going to these homes are Federal dollars, and the statutes clearly establish the Federal responsibility to assure that these funds go to services meeting standards, then disgraces in these homes may well lead to accusations of Federal non-feasance. We have already seen instances in studies by the Senate Committee on Aging, the Senate Finance Committee and by Ralph Nader.

The president chose to implement "Option Five," which, in the words of Richardson, "would give the Administration the initiative in this politically sensitive field and enable us to be on the offensive rather than reacting defensively to continuing criticism." The plan called for the training of 2,000 state inspectors, for the establishment of an Office of Nursing Home Affairs to coordinate enforcement activities, the hiring of 142 new people in HEW, the training of 20,000 nursing home personnel, the federal government's paying 100 percent of the cost of state inspections for two years, and the funding of "ombudsmen" units in five states to receive and investigate nursing home complaints.

Undersecretary John Veneman explained this plan to the subcommittee, indicating that the president was deeply committed to nursing home reform and that HEW was up to the task. He acknowledged the GAO study which showed that 50 percent of the homes in three states did not meet standards, and added that according to HEW studies, some states would have an even higher rate of noncompliance. His explanation was, "Reliance on State enforcement machinery has led to widespread non-enforcement of standards." However, under close questioning, the undersecretary admitted that the Nixon "reforms" would still place primary responsibility for the enforcement of federal standards in the hands of the states.

Appearing at the 1971 White House Conference on Aging, Secretary Richardson gave the impression that the power given to the secretary by the 1967 Moss amendments might be used. He threatened to cut off funds to 39 states that were out of compliance with Medicaid certification procedures. This threat resulted in the primary positive result of the Nixon "reforms": states began using federal criteria to certify homes for Medicaid and Medicare instead of simply certifying those homes which met state licensure standards.

In reality, however, the Nixon nursing home "reforms" amounted to little. For all the publicity, few homes were closed. Of the more than 7,000 Medicaid skilled nursing homes, 327—or less than 5 percent— left the program, 202 voluntarily. Secretary Richardson told the 1971 White House Conference on Aging that HEW had decertified 100 homes participating in Medicare. Thereafter, Reverend John Mason, director of social services for the American Lutheran Church, wrote to the secretary:

> The quality of your inspection and enforcement program is not something I would be proud of in my program. If 6,500 homes have participated in Medicare at one time or another and HEW has decertified 100 and perhaps another 43 now hanging in abeyance, that means about 1.5 percent have been disqualified for failure to meet standards.

In an effort to get a more objective analysis of the success of the Nixon "reforms," Senator Moss sent a questionnaire to 150 long term care experts representing every medical and health discipline, as well as senior citizen and consumer organizations. Some 120 returns were received, and 101 indicated that the president's plan had not reached the major problems in the field of long term care. Asked "has the quality of patient care been improved by the Nixon 'reforms'?" 63 percent said to a minor degree; 18 percent said not at all; 17 percent felt there has been substantial improvement. Asked to describe their overall opinion of the president's commitment to nursing home reform, most of the comments were negative. One expert said, "I emphasize the President's political motivations in his eight point program for nursing homes." A second said, "the President mouths pious words but does little to reach the real problems involved, namely financing of institutional care." Another added, "Viewed in its totality, six of the eight

points are generally punitive, vindictive, punishing, threatening, op-
pressive and negative." Yet another said it was a "well meaning but
misdirected flop."

In more recent days, HEW has shown greater attention to
reorganizing authority structures within the department than to the
serious business of seeing that standards were enforced.
Undersecretary Frank Carlucci announced Phase II of the department's nursing home reforms in 1974. Like its Nixon predecessor, it
amounted to little. The primary merit of the plan lay in its detailed
study of some 300 nursing homes and its stout defense of the stricter
regulations suggested in the Kennedy amendment.

Under pressure from Senators Moss and Kennedy, HEW had issued
new regulations for licensing administrators more in keeping with congressional intent. The new regulations prohibited domination of the
boards by the industry or its surrogates. These new regulations were
immediately challenged by a coalition of nursing home interests. With
urging from the Senate sponsors, HEW successfully defended the
regulations and won the suit, and as of 1977 all states were reported in
compliance.

Even if the Nixon "reforms" had been implemented in full, the
simple fact remains that states still have the exclusive responsibility
enforcement. Federal personnel will still spend their time shuffling
papers and shepherding state surveyors and enforcement personnel.
This fact remains even though, as Secretary Richardson warned the
president, "the statutes clearly establish Federal responsibility to
assure that funds go to services meeting standards." What should be
obvious is that when 50 states set out to enforce federal standards,
there will be great variations in the kind and degree of enforcement.
Since the responsibility for enforcement of federal standards is
superimposed on a system which is generally ineffective (even in the
enforcement of state standards), it should be clear that once again the
"reliance of State enforcement machinery will lead to widespread non-
enforcement of standards."

WHY STATE ENFORCEMENT SYSTEMS ARE INEFFECTIVE

Having established that much of the responsibility for the lax enforcement of nursing home standards lies with the federal government, a closer look at these procedures is in order. What follows is a
documentation of why Governor David Pryor, a former Arkansas congressman, called nursing home inspections "a national farce," why the
lieutenant governor of Wisconsin concluded the system was totally un-

workable, and why the state panel investigating the Baltimore salmonella deaths concluded the inspection and enforcement system was much to blame for the tragedy.

Fragmented Responsibility

Even if the federal government is successful in solving the serious problem of fragmentation at the federal level, this serious problem will remain to haunt the states which actually undertake inspection and enforcement. In most states the present system means that one agency licenses and inspects nursing homes, another pays the nursing home, and often, a third will assign patients to the facilities. In most states, if there is a formal effort to close a home, a fourth agency is brought in. This often leads to the situation in which one agency is trying to close a home while another is placing patients in it.

At the same time, there is fragmentation along political lines. Most states have four components to their inspection systems: sanitation and environment, meals, fire safety, and patient care. Thus, the annual inspection required by most states will not be complete until there has been a visit from a sanitarian, a dietician, a professional review team, and a fire inspector, who often appear at different times to look at different parts of the package. Yet another possible complication is duplication of effort by city, county, and state governments.

A study in Wisconsin showed that the separate agencies involved barely had any communication with one another. The filing system was in shambles. Sanitarians' and engineers' inspections reports were in one file cabinet and nurse inspectors' reports were in another, with no attempt to coordinate the two. Inspection forms were duplicated, various sections of the law were misapplied, and the information on many nursing homes was lost.

Infrequent Inspections

While some homes may be overinspected, subcommittee data confirm that most homes are underinspected. In Wisconsin, the lieutenant governor's report stressed that homes are not inspected annually as required by law. Of the 99 nursing homes in Milwaukee County, 34 had gone from 13 to 36 months without being inspected. Infrequent inspections were noted by the Maryland investigatory panel, and the director of the Illinois Department of Health explained away the fact that 50 percent of the nursing homes in his state did not meet standards by saying, "I guess we weren't in there often enough."

Many health officers will readily admit inspections are infrequent and blame this on the inadequate numbers of personnel. In Minnesota, Dr. Warren Lawson testified that the 1941 licensing law authorized two inspectors and one clerk in that state. Thirty years later there were still only two inspectors and one clerk, even though the number of nursing home patients had increased from 4,000 to 41,000.

Advance Notice of Inspections

The subcommittee documented sufficient evidence of the practice of giving advance notice to warn operators of pending inspections to believe it is a widespread national problem. The practice was documented in Florida, Minnesota, Illinois, Wisconsin, and Maryland. There is little doubt that this practice vitiates the effectiveness of the inspection and enforcement process. During the Minnesota hearing, one LPN testified:

> This home always knew in advance whenever the health department was due to come out for an inspection. Consequently, they could put extra work in and clean the place up and make it look good before they came. They would also get people from other shifts to be on duty when the inspector was there so it looked like they were not understaffed. That way it would look like they had a full staff when they really didn't.

Another witness testified:

> When the health inspectors come, the home is notified. When Margaret Christianson is going to inspect, she notifies them every time. She writes them a letter or calls at least 3 or 4 days ahead of time. When the home finds out, everybody rushes around cleaning up, and they have everything spic and span when the inspector comes. One time one of the registered nurses told me to move some cleaning fluid, which was poison, from a floor cabinet to up high because Christianson was coming. I said, "How do you know?" and she said, "She called."

Inspections as Bureaucratic Rituals

Inspections in many states, with or without the benefit of prior announcement, tend to be cursory or pro forma. The Maryland panel investigating the epidemic concluded:

It has become evident from this investigation that mechanisms for licensing and inspection of nursing homes, while superficially appearing thorough and penetrating, are inadequate in Maryland.

While on paper the rules for licensure and the criteria for inspection seem reasonable and thorough, there was abundant evidence at the hearings (on the salmonella deaths) that inspections were infrequent, that nursing homes generally knew when they were to take place, that inspection reports were sometimes in conflict with one another, and that violations almost never resulted in revocation of licensure.

Indeed our panel felt at certain points in the testimony that inspections were a bureaucratic ritual carried out in a fashion which led to a tidy series of papers which were duly filed as evidence of accomplishment rather than signals for action.

Relationships Between the Regulator and the Regulated

Almost inevitably, nursing home surveyors become friends with certain nursing home administrators and as a result might have a tendency to be lax in their enforcement of standards with the favored facility. Conversely, they can be very tough if they dislike an administrator. While this is only human nature, the practice is helped along by some operators who offer bribes and gratuities. The practice is also encouraged by procedures which give surveyors discretion not to report each and every violation.

Inspectors' Recommendations Are Ignored

The unfortunate practice in many states is to ignore the findings and recommendations of state surveyors. There are ample examples in subcommittee files of inspectors bringing abuses to the attention of their superiors, with no results. Homes not recommended for relicensure have been routinely relicensed — even those guilty of serious protracted violations. Inspectors with the temerity to complain to the newspapers or to the subcommittee were "disciplined" by their superiors for "making trouble." The subcommittee's experience, especially in Minnesota, Wisconsin, and Illinois, documents these conclusions.

In Illinois, Bill Recktenwald, chief investigator of the Chicago Better Government Association testified to the "callous neglect by state officials in seeking any kind of reform." With investigator Bill Hood, he provided these examples from Illinois state health files:

• Largent's Nursing Home is located south of suburban Midlothian. This home, operated by a woman who is herself confined to a wheel chair, first came under criticism from health inspectors in 1950. State files show that Largent's was repeatedly found in violation of nursing homes codes for the next 10 years.

Nevertheless, its license was never revoked, although inspectors had recommended such action numerous times.

In March 1967, this home was found in violation of 14 codes and was not recommended for relicensure.

It was then given 10 follow-up inspections over a period of 3 years, in an effort to get a passing grade from health inspectors. Its license was finally revoked, and it lost its status as a nursing home. One month later, the license was reinstated, with no record that the owner had corrected a single violation.

• In each of the last 5 years, inspectors have recommended the Burr Oak Nursing and Convalescent Center be closed.

In 1966, the food service was so bad the chief nutritionist of Cook County Department of Public Health asked no license be given. A 1967 survey team found a "complete and utter disregard for good patient care in this facility." The report listed 29 violations and the entire team vetoed relicensing. In 1968, the fire marshal found serious violations and ordered immediate corrections.

The 1969 visit to this 38-bed facility, although announced beforehand, found diet orders for patients completely lacking, dirty food storage areas and the patients' medical record book was missing.

The three-man team investigating in 1970 found:

1. No one in charge of the patients when they arrived.
2. The condition of the patients was described as "very unclean, feet badly in need of washing and the skin on the feet was dirty and hard."
3. Patients' rooms were dirty, disorderly, and floors throughout the home were unclean.
4. There was a "strong urine odor throughout the home."
5. Medicine distribution very bad and records of who got what could not be found.

In sum, the place was not recommended for relicensure. The Cook County Department of Public Health called it one of its worse homes. It is still in business today.

• The Styrest Nursing Home in Carbondale has had many complaints and bad reports through the years. State files revealed that two residents died under odd circumstances. One patient, found by a family member, was tied in a chair while running a 106° temperature. She died the next day. The other patient was reportedly found starving and dehydrated by a member of the family. She also died the day after she was found.

The entire nursing staff submitted a list of grievances to the administrator in 1970. A copy was filed with the state. The nurses complained of:

1. skeletal nursing staff,
2. obligations to patients not met,
3. skilled home standards not met,
4. diabetic patients' insulin reactions due to home's poorly calculated diet.
5. patients clothing and personal funds not being used properly, and
6. neglect of some very ill patients.

Despite the above complaints and an additional complaint from the editor of a weekly paper in Carbondale, a renewed license was granted in March of this year without any evidence that the complaints had been investigated or that conditions had changed.

These reports from state health department files were confirmed by the inspectors themselves. For many years, Cook County Department of Health, which had power to inspect but not to close homes, had been calling such matters to the attention of the state with no results. In desperation, they testified before the subcommittee. As a result, the Cook County Department of Public Health was stripped of all enforcement responsibilities by the state. This is true even though the hearings documented that the inspectors had been doing the most effective job in the state. Clearly, an embarrassed state retaliated against the county officials.

In Milwaukee, two nursing home inspectors had to file an appeal in circuit court to get the State Department of Health and Social Services to restore satisfactory ratings to their personnel files. Although they had excellent records in the past, the two inspectors were given unsatisfactory ratings and denied merit increases after the *Milwaukee Sentinel* carried a series of articles on nursing home conditions. The *Sentinel* charged that 43 out of 99 homes in Milwaukee County had serious violations that jeopardized patient safety. The lieutenant governor's report confirmed the *Milwaukee Sentinel* story. The computer study showed that 51 out of 99 homes in the county had serious violations.

Political Influence Keeps Some Homes Open

The subcommittee's investigtion of the files of several state health departments revealed many cases in which political influence kept nursing homes from being disciplined. Often, letters were couched in the mildest terms, but the interest of a powerful state senator or other official was enough to cause the state to mollify its criticism of a home or to ignore violations. The Chicago hearings provided these examples:

> • The 69 bed Rosary Nursing Home in Tinley Park has had consistently bad reports for the past 4 years. Most inspectors have recommended the place be closed but it has remained open.
> It appears political pressure was applied in 1968. A memo found in Illinois files from inspector F.H. Williams to the coordinator of the Licensure and Certification section mentions the "political implications involved."
> These implications apparently stem from queries by State Representative Walter "Babe" McAvoy to Dr. Yoder, head of the Department of Public Health, in regard to the Rosary Nursing Home. A license was issued in that year.
> In the following 2 years, 1969, and 1970, inspectors again found conditions bad and recommended no relicensure. The home remains open today.

> • Palos Hills Convalescent Center, in Palos Hills, and Whitehaven Acres in Glenview are both owned in substantial part by one Frank Williams, former president of the Illinois Nursing Home Association. Both these homes have been severely criticized by inspectors. Recommendations have been made that both lose their licenses. These repeated pleas have been ignored.

The attitude of the owner, Mr. Frank Williams, has been part of the problem. A State inspector wrote the following paragraph to his superiors in Springfield in April 1969, and I quote: "I have been reliably informed, and his actions further bear out the fact, that Mr. Williams feels that he, in his position, is above the law, and feels that his homes should be overlooked. ... The Whitehaven Acres Nursing Home is one of the most substandard homes that I have seen."*

The Permissive Attitude of Many State Health Departments

Many state health departments take a permissive attitude towards the nursing homes in their state. Vigorous enforcement of standards creates only problems for them. First and foremost is the problem of where to put the patients who would be dispossessed if homes were closed. It is also noteworthy that enforcement costs money, most of which would come out of the budget of the health department. These two factors and the lack of any legal alternative short of closure causes many state health departments to adopt a " give them another chance" policy. In Milwaukee, for example, the lieutenant governor found that it was quite common for the state to give violators grace periods of 40 to 44 weeks to come into compliance. There was no limit on the length of time a home could be given to meet requisite standards.

Most health departments believe that fines are relatively ineffective in prohibiting abuses and that the cumbersome administrative or legal procedures involved in closing a home make the effort counterproductive. They feel that judges have a bias against depriving the operator of a livelihood, particularly if the operator shows that the matters have been or will be corrected. Dr. Bruce Flashner, deputy director of the Illinois Department of Health testified:

The other thing: every time a proceeding went to court, it got either thrown out, or somebody found some reason for delaying any action, so that is a sense, the department, which should not be absolved from blame, got more blame than it deserved.

You cannot do anything unless the courts are going to back you.

The absence of other enforcement tools is a major reason that so many homes are substandard today. The health department can expect

---

*See Chapter 11 for more examples.

that any unilateral action it takes will be challenged in court by the industry. Suits have been brought challenging the right of the state to remove patients placed in a particular home by a state agency or challenging the state's right to cut off payment of public assistance funds. Every state statute is different: some provide for injunction relief which can be brought only in extraordinary cases, when the state can show immediate or irreparable injury. Attempts are under way in several states to provide alternatives to the formal, legal procedure of closing the nursing home.

Why are so few homes closed? The basic reason is that the state is not prepared to deal with the relocation of patients. "Where will we put them?" was the common cry by state officials. Administrators' refusal to take welfare patients compounds the problem. In short, they rationalize that a poor nursing home is a better place for these people than the street. Kenneth C. Eymann, editor of *Professional Nursing Homes*, commented in the September 1964 issue, "This is about the same as saying if you are starving to death, even poison is better nourishment than nothing at all! In these enlightened times it is appalling that such a philosophy can exist."

The Illinois Department of Health testified that places could probably be found if it decided to close down perhaps five percent of its nursing home beds. But the decision to close a home is more complicated. The 1970 Report to the Governor of Michigan on Nursing Home Problems states the problem:

> This enforced wholesale movement of patients can cause great inconvenience and actual physical harm to these patients. Thus, revocation of license adversely affects the very people the government seeks to secure. For this reason alone, revocation of license must be used only in severe situations when correction of facility inadequacies is demonstrably not forthcoming and the potential harm to the patients caused by enforced transfer is less than the potential harm to the patients if allowed to stay in the facility persisting in those uncorrected deficiencies.

This comment provides good perspective. States need enforcement tools short of formal legal procedures, which are protracted and expensive. The closing of a home should be a last resort, after all reasonable efforts have been made to help bring about compliance. In the face of recurrent violations, substandard facilities must be closed. To allow the operation of substandard facilities causes other caretakers not to take the regulations seriously. Perhaps more important, substandard homes have a competitive advantage over the good faith operator. By not meeting standards they can maximize profit.

Conclusion

The fact that 50 percent of the nursing homes in the U.S. are substandard and that so few homes are closed adequately points up the shortcomings of the enforcement system and the measure of HEW's default. It is abundantly evident that the federal government cannot and should not rely totally upon state enforcement machinery.

Chapter 11

Political Influence and The Nursing Home

In the summer of 1974, the city of New York virtually exploded in the wake of a newspaper exposé about nursing homes written by *New York Times* writer, John Hess. It was no ordinary exposé dealing with surface issues, but then John Hess is no ordinary reporter, and the *New York Times* is no ordinary newspaper.

Mr. Hess was aided in his efforts by the interest of a young assemblyman, Andrew Stein, chairman of what was called the Temporary Commission on Living Costs and the Environment. Andy Stein's investigators had plenty of company in the field. Bill Cabin from the New York Welfare Inspector General's Office had been conducting an audit of the 347-bed Towers Nursing Home owned by Rabbi Bernard Bergman. Cabin's preliminary report set off more shock waves. All of the New York press corps, including veterans like Jack Newfield of *The Village Voice* and Steve Bauman of WNEW-TV, joined the chase investigating New York's nursing home millionnaires.

The public's imagination was soon captured by Mr. Bergman, who in a short time had built himself a $24 million nursing home and a related real estate empire largely out of Medicaid funds. What made the Bergman case unique was not the many allegations of poor care and abuse nor the fact that $2.2 million could not be accounted for in the Towers loan and exchange account. It was not the fact that Bergman's accountant, Samuel Dachowitz had deposited some $807,000 in checks from the Towers Nursing Home in his private account, nor was it the fact that Medicaid funds were used to furnish Towers administrator, Mark Loren, with a Chrysler automobile and other amenities.[1] What made the Bergman case unique was the revelation of the involvement of New York's major political figures with nursing homes. New Yorkers, and most of the nation, were shocked to learn of the extent to which politicians used their influence to benefit nursing home interests.

The Subcommittee on Long Term Care investigated these matters, issuing over 60 subpoenas to nursing home operators, vendors, and banks. Mr. Bergman was ordered to appear before the subcommittee on January 21, 1975. At that time, he produced his books and records for the subcommittee and declared that he was an innocent victim of a vendetta perpetrated by state officials and the media which "had no parallel in modern history since the days of Senator Joseph McCarthy."

Mr. Bergman bristled noticeably under a line of questioning related to his political contacts. He claimed the appeals to politicians were proper and necessary to cut through red tape and bureaucratic bungling. Asked if he had ever requested Stanley Steingut, speaker of the New York State Assembly to arrange a meeting with then Governor Nelson Rockefeller, he first responded that he had no knowledge of events. It was suggested to him that such a conversation might have taken place at his daughter's wedding.

"I was too excited and busy to remember whether I had such a conversation," said Bergman. He later admitted that such a meeting had taken place in the governor's New York City office. But the details of who attended the meeting and what the purpose of it was were never clarified.

The subcommittee asked Bergman to return on February 4, 1975. By that time, Bergman's books and records would have been analyzed, and specific questions could be asked. Despite his promise, Bergman failed to appear at the second hearing. His lawyer argued that the witness was not required to be present. The subcommittee members contended the opposite, claiming that the terms of the January 21 subpoena carried over.

Meeting in Washington later, the full Senate Committee on Aging met to discuss Bergman's failure to comply. A decision was made to hold the contempt citation in abeyance and to give Mr. Bergman one more chance to appear, this time before the full committee.

On February 17, 1975, Bergman did appear before the committee, but he asserted his constitutional rights against self-incrimination. His attorney made note of the fact that Mr. Bergman was facing possible criminal charges being considered at that time by Charles J. Hynes, special prosecutor for nursing homes, state of New York.

Accordingly, it remained for New York's Moreland Act Commission on Nursing Homes and Residential Facilities to complete the probe into political influence and related issues. Under the direction of Morris

B. Abram, the commission produced a report, "Political Influence and Political Accountability: One Foot in the Door." The report stands as a classic description of the process which takes place (albeit on a smaller scale) in almost every state. A review of the facts in that report provides a sobering lesson and shows that political influence is an important reason for the continuing nursing home abuses.

In our investigations we learned that most commonly operators prevail upon politicians to prevent sanctions from being applied against their homes. Politicians are often asked to help extend a deadline for compliance with standards or to prevent the closing of a home for its failure to conform to fire safety standards. A Texas state senator recently called an inspector to tell him that he (the senator) would be present at a certain facility at the time of the inspection "just to make sure that it was done right." In Wisconsin, an office holder intervened with senior health department officials to stifle recommendations for discipline that were filed by inspectors. In California, one official wrote to the chief inspector for Los Angeles County reminding the inspector that a particular operator was a good friend of his and warned the inspector against taking any action against the nursing home without notifying the legislator first.

Another type of abuse of political power is obtaining preferences for nursing home operators. For example, politicians have arranged for the appointment of nursing home representatives to various licensure or planning boards in exchange for political contributions or the delivery of votes. Special bills are sometimes pushed through state legislatures to benefit owners. In one case, a special bill was quietly eased through the Minnesota legislature to circumvent an ordinance prohibiting the building of a nursing home within 300 feet of a flammable liquids storage depot (several state legislators had a financial interest in the home).

There have even been cases in which elected representatives have been induced to conduct "friendly" investigations of nursing home interests. In at least one instance, the expenses for these bogus hearings were absorbed by nursing home representatives. To complete the "white wash," elected officials have issued reports proclaiming their state free from any serious nursing home problems. At times, they have denounced state officials for "overzealous" reform efforts.

Still other abuses involve legislators representing nursing homes before state rate setting or other regulatory agencies. In this situation, the public may rightly wonder whether the legislator is functioning in his private or public capacity.

As the Moreland Act Commission noted, the central issue in New York appeared to be Mr. Bergman's efforts to secure a license for the 240-bed Danube Nursing Home built in Staten Island without a certificate of need. Bergman's involvement reads like a novel of political intrigue, its list of characters like a *Who's Who* of New York politics. Among the more than one dozen major political figures charged with political interference, negligence, and impropriety were former Governors Nelson A. Rockefeller and Malcom Wilson, Attorney General Louis J. Lefkowitz, Assembly Speaker Stanley Steingut, New York Mayor Abraham Beame, and Robert Patton, second deputy commissioner of the New York State Department of Mental Hygiene.

The Moreland Commission report (which provides the basis for the forthcoming conclusions in this chapter) says that Bergman's technique was to harness himself to people involved with the "acquistion and exercise of political power." His major source of strength "was his close alliance with Samuel Hausman," a close associate and political advisor of Governor Rockefeller. Bergman got Hausman's help by "grossly misusing the deference paid to him [Bergman] as a prominent leader in the Orthodox Jewish community and by granting commercial favors to a Hausman relative." The report states:

> Hausman, who served as the Governor's informal "eyes and ears to the Jewish Community" sought to control access to the Executive Chamber with respect to matters of significance to the Jewish Community and to convert the access which he granted to representatives of this largely Democratic group of voters to the advantage of the Rockefeller and Wilson administrations. Bergman, perceiving Hausman's importance, exploited it for his own financial gain. With Hausman reveling in his expeditor's role on Bergman's behalf, Bergman and his associates were able to secure easy access to all levels of state government from the Chiefs of Staff and Secretaries to Governors Rockefeller and Wilson, down to commissioners, deputy commissioners and lower level officials at several different state agencies, achieving as a consequence important favorable decisions.

Hausman admitted that he did intervene on Bergman's behalf a great number of times in arranging meetings with some of the most powerful men in America, including Robert Douglass, Rockefeller's secretary, in 1971 and later with his successor, T. Norman Hurd. He also arranged meetings with Governor Malcolm Wilson, who succeeded Rockefeller.

Clearly, the place that Hausman could help Bergman the most was the governor's mansion. The principal door opener for Hausman (and thus for Bergman) was T. Norman Hurd, secretary to Governors Rockefeller and Wilson. In the words of the commission, Hurd "devoted substantial amounts of time and effort assisting Bergman in getting some state agency to make use of an empty nursing home which Bergman had illegally constructed." The commission added, "The only plausible explanation for Hurd's activity was his desire to please Hausman, a man of importance to Rockefeller and thereafter Wilson."

Hurd admitted that he met with Hausman and Bergman about a dozen times from 1972 through 1974 to discuss the Danube home. The alleged result of one of those visits was the so-called April 1, 1974 secret agreement signed by Robert Patton. Patton testified that Hurd called his boss, director of the State Department of Mental Hygiene to arrange for the transfer of patients to the Bergman home.

The long and the short of it is that Bergman and his son-in-law, Amram Kaas, did everything possible to obtain a license for the nursing home they constructed without a certificate of need. They hired lawyers Deputy Mayor Stanley Lowell, State Senator John Marchi, and C. Daniel Chill, legislative assistant to Speaker Steingut to represent them. They met with an brought pressure to bear on state health department employees. For example, Chill wrote to Andrew Fleck, first deputy commissioner of health, on Bergman's behalf, using official stationery from the speaker's office but typing "personal and unofficial" at the bottom of it. When they were turned down, they decided to go the political route—to make an end run around resisting state health department officials. After meeting with Hurd and then Governor Wilson, they finally got what they wanted—a secret agreement to move hundreds of mentally retarded patients from Willowbrook to the Bergman facility.

But the secret agreement did not stay secret very long. The discovery of the details generated a tremendous public protest. The Staten Island Community Organization protested the move and ultimately was successful in stopping the transfer. But it was an uphill fight.

State Senator John Marchi found himself in an uncomfortable position, to say the least. He had been representing Bergman's son-in-law in the Danube matter, and his constituency was apparently violently opposed to the project he was backing.

Sonia Braniff, the mother of a handicapped daughter, was in the forefront of the battle to stop the transfer of the patients, and she really felt the pressure. She served as president of her local United Cerebral Palsy chapter. She testified that she received a telephone call from the main office in New York City about her position in the Danube matter. New York officers pointed out to her that Samuel Hausman, a man of considerable influence and wealth and one of the founders of the organization, was "interested" in the project. She was further reminded that Hausman's brother, Leo, was chairman of the board of that organization.

Hausman was apparently oblivious to the conflict of interest in his dual role as a lobbyist for Bergman and as a member of the State Hospital Review and Planning Council and the State Medical Care Facilities Finance Agency, charged the commission. He served on those two agencies as a Rockefeller appointee. Hausman explained he was only trying to help Bergman because Bergman had complained of discrimination against him (on the basis of his Orthodox Jewish religion) by state health department employees. "He duped and used me," said Hausman.

The Moreland Commission hearings provided additional details on the following New York politicians:

- *Assembly Speaker Steingut*, who had holdings in an insurance company called Grand Brokerage, along with Brooklyn Democratic boss, Meade Esposito, insured several Bergman-owned or controlled facilities. In testimony before the Moreland Commission he admitted intervening on Bergman's behalf three times—once to set up a meeting with Bergman and New York City Mayor Abraham Beame, once to set up a meeting with Governor Rockefeller and Bergman (the meeting was aborted when Rockefeller kept Steingut waiting and then refused to see him), and once with Assemblyman Andrew Stein's father for the purpose of getting Bergman's appearance before the Stein Commission postponed. Steingut admitted twelve meetings with Bergman in the years 1971-1974, but said only one related to nursing home business.
- *Mayor Abraham Beame* admitted meeting with Bergman twice on the Danube matter but told Bergman there was nothing he could do to help. He admitted receiving campaign contributions of

$20,000 from nursing home interests and another $25,000 loan during a mayorality race but asserted he had not given any favors in return.

- *State Senate Majority Leader Warren M. Anderson* served as counsel for several nursing homes.
- *Attorney General Louis Lefkowitz* was severely criticized by the commission for his close connections with voluntary nonprofit nursing homes. The commission offered as evidence several letters in which Lefkowitz sought and received increases in allowable costs for nursing home projects funded by the state of New York. He was also criticized for his failure to investigate nursing home abuses, and, it was noted, he had received a campaign contribution from Mr. Bergman.
- *Assistant Commissioner Al Schwartz of the New York City Health Department* was criticized for this "coziness" with nursing home operators as evidenced by his "destruction of critical inspection reports and his insistence on replacing them with 'love letters.' "
- *Assemblymen James L. Emery and Martin Ginzberg* apparently applied a great deal of pressure on health department officials in order to obtain preferential treatment for the nursing home interests they represented. Dr. Fleck kept meticulous records of every political demand made upon him. In this connection he wrote that "Emery was quite candid with me in indicating that he, along with Assemblyman Ginzberg, represented the interest of Mr. Al Schwartzberg," president of Di-Com Construction Company, a firm that specializes in the building of nursing homes.
- *Governor Nelson Rockefeller* was "cleared" of any wrongdoing in connection with nursing home problems by Assemblyman Andrew Stein. The Moreland Commission, however, came down heavily on the former governor. The commission stated that "Mr. Hurd and former Governors Rockefeller and Wilson regarded repeated interventions as 'mere courtesies' and denied that they had any intimidating effect on civil servants." The commission observed:

The Commission believes that such an attitude completely overlooks the subtleties and refinements by which subtle politicians manipulate decisions without appearing to do so. It also ignores the demoralizing effect which the perception of political influence has on public confidence in government.

The man in the best position to see the full scope and dimension of political influence and its effect on civil servants was Dr. Andrew Fleck. His files reveal contact after contact: telephone calls, letters, and even personal visits from office holders asking for preferential treatment for nursing homes. Dr. Fleck said the pressure came from every direction and from both political parties. He called the Danube situation a rape of New York public health laws. Asked who was responsible, he said that it was a gang rape.

One thing seems clear—the fraud and abuse in New York nursing homes could not have continued unabated for ten years without either the tacit support or inaction by elected public officials. The lesson is obvious.

Rabbi Bernard Bergman pleaded guilty to fraud on March 11, 1976 and was sentenced to one year in jail on September 15, 1976. He has been ordered to repay almost $2 million. Samuel Dachowitz was sentenced to one year and one day in jail and fined $17,500. Mark Loren received a three-month sentence and a $7,500 fine for his part in the conspiracy to defraud the government. Special Prosecutor Charles J. Hynes has issued over 100 indictments, obtained over 27 convictions, and identified more than $70 million in fraud or overpayments to nursing homes in New York since the subcommittee's January 1975 hearings. While many organizations and individuals should be credited for the progress that has been made with nursing homes in New York, the greater part of that credit belongs to the *New York Times* and to John Hess.

Chapter 12

The Physician's Abdication of Responsibility

Historically, physicians have abdicated their responsibility for nursing home patients. With the exception of a small minority, they are infrequent visitors to nursing homes. Sixteen years ago, the Subcommittee on Problems of the Aged and Aging of the Senate Committee on Labor and Public Affairs issued a report that concluded: "Management of patients in nursing homes by physicians is either lacking or inadequate."

Five years later, in 1965, Lillian B. McCall, consultant to the Ways and Means Committee of the California Assembly testified, "The Medical profession has turned its back on the aged. . . (the old age assistance program) has accelerated the entire program of segregating aged people, and I would say in a rather flat way that it is a medical care program in name only."

The 1969-76 series of subcommittee hearings proved that these observations are all the more valid today. Dr. Charles Kramer, president of the Kramer Foundation, clinical director of the Plum Grove Nursing Home, and Assistant Professor of Psychiatry, Univeristy of Illinois College of Medicine, reported that doctors pop in and out of nursing homes, that they seldom do more than make notations on charts. Dr. Dora Nicholson of Washington, D.C. testified to the great difficulty she encountered in obtaining medical care for her mother, a patient in a Maryland nursing home. She emphasized that she had money enough to hire the best specialists but was unable to get them to provide care. She concluded that if she had so much trouble, the average American must find it impossible. Dr. Lionel Z. Cousin said that the whole system of health care in America seems to be ill designed for the aged, adding that the average patient is better off in England than in America because of the American medical community's lack of interest in problems of the aged.

171

Why do physicians avoid nursing home patients? There are a number of reasons, ranging from inconvenience to inadequate reimbursement. Much of the problem is the lack of emphasis on the care of the aged in this country's schools of medicine. Many doctors avoid nursing homes because they get too depressed, simply reflecting the values of the youth-oriented American society, preferring the young to the old, the "curable" to the chronically ill.

REASONS FOR THE ABDICATION

The Shortage of Physicians

The U.S. Department of Labor estimated in 1972 that the United States was short some 50,000 physicians. Clearly, this shortage is compounded by a maldistribution of doctors who tend to centralize in large cities on the east and west coast, leaving rural areas hard-pressed for medical care.

What this means is that when the physician divides time among all the people, the elderly lose out. Physicians tend to feel their time is better spent with those members of society who have the most life before them.

Medical Schools' Failure to Emphasize Geriatrics

For all the specialization that has taken place in America, the practice of geriatrics has received little or no attention in U.S. medical schools. Surprising as it seems, most medical students graduate without understanding the special medical problems of the elderly. For example, the elderly often should not be given the same strength and quantities of drugs as younger Americans. This is true because older Americans have:

- reduced metabolic activity necessitating lower doses;
- an altered response of the central nervous system so that confusion is often associated with sedation;
- a reduced rate of elimination so that the drugs are retained in the body longer, which can lead to overdoses;
- impairment of the homeostatic mechanism;
- greater variability in response to drugs than younger Americans.

The degree to which the study of geriatrics has been neglected was emphasized by the results of a subcommittee questionnaire sent to all of this nation's 104 schools of medicine in 1971. Only three schools indicated that they would soon implement an area of specialization or create a department of geriatrics.

Only six schools reported having programs whereby students worked with nursing homes. Seven schools indicated they served nursing homes in some other way, largely by providing consultants in some capacity. One school reported students were serving nursing homes as "externs," apparently a reference to the fact that nursing homes are often a source of employment for moonlighting interns.

Typical of the response received by the committee is the following letter from Dean David E. Rodgers of the Johns Hopkins University School of Medicine. It should be added that Dr. Rodgers is a good deal more candid in the terms with which he answered the questionnaire. Most deans went to great pains to tell the committee that they included geriatrics in a more general course on human development or cited the school's gerontological research programs. Dr. Rodgers wrote:

October 25, 1971

Senator Frank E. Moss
United States Senate
Washington, D.C. 20510

Dear Senator Moss:

I'm afraid, as with most medical schools, we do a thoroughly inadequate job in all the areas that you questioned me about. Despite being a member of a committee that examined a catastrophe in a nursing home here in Baltimore, the answer to all three of your questions is "no." More specifically:

1. No, we do not have geriatrics as a speciality in our curriculum.
2. We do not have programs in which students, interns or residents serve in nursing homes.
3. We have virtually no contact with the elderly who are in nursing homes — though we are currently exploring ways of developing some kind of program for students which will get them acquainted with the problems of the forgotten — our aging sick.

I firmly believe that all these areas are of increasing importance to us — and this school, as well as many others, should be involved in it.

Sincerely yours,
/s/ David E. Rodgers
David E. Rodgers, M.D.
Dean of the Medical Faculty

In 1974, a second questionnaire was sent. Although some increased interest in the problems of the aged was demonstrated by the 100 schools responding, the results were still far from encouraging. Thirteen percent indicated their program now included or alternatively was in the process of including geriatrics as a specialty. Twenty-six percent said they now had a program whereby students could fulfill requirements by serving in nursing homes.

In 1976, a third questionnaire was sent. The result was a regression from the 1974 results. Only ten schools indicated that they had or were contemplating the establishment of a chair in geriatric medicine or otherwise would give geriatrics special attention.

The Ineffective Administration of Medicare and Medicaid

Another factor which explains the absence of the physician from the nursing home setting is the quixotic administration of Medicare and Medicaid. The red tape and changing rules of these two programs constitute a significant disincentive for physicians to visit nursing home patients. The basic problem of inadequate compensation is compounded by the uncertainty of payment. Clerks in insurance offices who never see patients overrule the judgment of physicians as to the eligibility of patients for payment, and physicians who submit large bills to Medicare and Medicaid are looked upon with suspicion.

Regulations Require Few Visits

The regulations in effect until January 1974 for both the Medicare and Medicaid programs required physicians to visit nursing home patients at least once every 30 days. That requirement was never enforced, as can be seen from the May 1971 GAO audit of three states, which found this requirement was violated in more than 50 percent of the homes surveyed.

In January 1974, new regulations were announced by HEW requiring physicians to see patients once every 30 days for the first three months, and at 60-day intervals thereafter, in effect diluting the standard and excusing doctors' absence from nursing homes. That patients need to see their physicians more rather than less frequently should be clear from the following, excerpted from a letter by Dr. J. Raymond Gladue, president of the American Association of Nursing Home Physicians:

> The Bureau of Health Insurance (Medicare) should know that chronically ill aged patients are less resistant to all forms of

stress, physical, psychological and emotional, and that therapy must be brought to bear quickly to prevent irreparable damage and/or death. Studies show that morbidity and mortality are favorably affected by frequency of physicians' visits. Are you aware that, from a physical standpoint, the bedridden or physically inactive chronically ill patient (who needn't even be old, but advanced age certainly doesn't help!) is always subject to, and must therefore be constantly watched for, a number of conditions:

- Heightened susceptibility to illness of any type, epidemic or otherwise, and the fact that even a minor cold or virus caught from an attendant or visitor could quickly and easily escalate into a major or fatal disease unless promptly noted and treated.
- Kidney diseases or other urinary difficulties.
- Bed sores, skin irritations, etc.
- Cardiac failure and irregularities of rhythm must be recognized early and treated promptly.
- Bowel difficulties which, unless watched and corrected, are far from minor problems to the patient.
- Dietary deficiencies which may be brought about by the patient's condition or because he, even though offered a proper diet, may for various reasons not eat as he should. Diseases of teeth and gums are often implicated.
- Changes which may occur in the effectiveness of medication, even though it may have been given over a long period of time without apparent difficulties. Such changes could be the result of changes in the patient's condition or of the fact that sometimes (many examples come to mind) effects are cumulative and difficulties take months or years to become apparent. Many medications are still too new to assume that everything is known about them.
- Changes in brain function, very common and resulting in confusion, disorientation and depression and/or agitation. These conditions can be treated effectively by the physician with the use of understanding, psychotherapy, and psycho-active drugs.
- Deterioration of vision and hearing. The physician must be alert to changes which can affect the patient's ability to communicate. Most are correctable or can be helped.

The Scarcity of Trained Personnel

In addition to the disincentives already mentioned, it is apparent that doctors do not have the back-up or support in a nursing home which they have come to expect in a hospital. Yet, as Dr. Gladue's letter indicates, the medical challenge is in many ways even greater.

It appears there is a widespread opinion among members of the medical profession that nursing home personnel are capable of providing only shoddy care. As a consequence of this attitude, patients are often referred to homes unsuitable to their needs or referred without adequate medical attention or with inadequate medical information. Dr. Victor Kassel summed up in his testimony:

> Doctors don't want to visit nursing homes for a number of reasons. Too many of the persons working there are incompetent. For example, a doctor takes time to visit a home and the person left in charge by the administrator isn't expecting him.
>
> Then, the aides have a hard time finding the patient's medical chart, or even the patient himself, since sometimes the aides don't know the names of the patients and are unable to direct the doctor to the individual he is to examine.
>
> When he finally locates the patient he sits down on a chair that has been urinated upon. Additionally, lighting in most nursing homes is made for seduction rather than for any kind of examination.
>
> Doctors dislike nursing home visits because everything is against them. It takes them ten times as long to accomplish anything.

Nursing Homes' Depressing and Unpleasant Atmosphere

Even physicians, supposedly calloused by years of dealing with the sick and helpless, admit experiencing depression when in a nursing home. Dr. Thomas H. Clark said:

> The nursing home can be a depressing place, especially if you are approaching nursing home age yourself. When you see these people, you think, "this is going to happen to me," and you unconsciously avoid nursing homes for this reason. And, too, with the elderly patient, it is easy to get frozen into a diagnosis, then to stop thinking about the patient anymore.

Dr. Kassel testified, "I hate to go to a nursing home. You do not want to sit down. You are afraid to touch things. Patients are confused, and they will wipe stool on the doorknob. The care of nursing home patients is a difficult job and you have to be very dedicated."

Distance Between the Office, the Hospital and the Nursing Home

Even those physicians who are inclined to visit nursing home patients may be discouraged by distance. For this reason, many physicians testified as to the desirability of locating nursing homes adjacent to or near to hospitals. At the present time, most nursing homes are free-standing, that is, isolated from hospitals, which often requires the physician to travel from 20 minutes to an hour to see patients. Under present rules, this typical visit would bring the physician less than $20. Any reasonable computation of what the physician's time is worth per hour proves that this is a strong disincentive to visiting nursing home patients.

The Marcus Welby Syndrome

As noted, the primary emphasis of medical education in the U.S. is acute illness. The acute hospital is the focus of the medical profession. The largest portion of the American health dollar goes to pay for hospital bills. Clearly, acute illness is more lucrative. But there is another reason that doctors have abdicated their responsibility for the infirm elderly. It grows out of ego pride, out of a desire to "cure" patients and receive the satisfactions that come from doing so.

Dr. Ewald Busse, director of the Center for the Study of Aging at Duke University, has written:

> There are few physicians who are capable of dealing with the large numbers of chronically ill persons with sustained enthusiasm .... The physician, like all other people, if he is to live and work effectively must maintain self-esteem. The physician's evaluation of himself as an individual capable of eliminating pain and restoring function is apt to suffer when he cannot see clearly the patient's improvement as a result of his efforts.[1]

In short, many physicians stay away from nursing home patients because they feel they are unable to heal them. Practicing geriatricians such as Dr. Cousin and Dr. Kassel call this a cruel fallacy.

Geriatric patients in nursing homes can be aided. Many of them can and have staged dramatic recoveries regaining power of speech or mobility. Because these facts are so often overlooked, Senator Moss labeled this rationalization for not visiting patients the "Marcus Welby Syndrome."

CONSEQUENCES OF THE ABDICATION

The clear result of the physician's abdication of responsibility for the elderly is poor care and the failure to meet the needs of the patient. The problems created fall into three categories: inattention to patients' needs, the lack of control on drugs, and the failure to report infectious diseases.

Inattention to the Needs of Patients

Several studies by nursing home professionals underscore the need for greater physician involvement. For example, a 1971 study by the Utah Nursing Home Association concluded: "It's almost impossible for the welfare patient to get medical care.... Dumping welfare patients is a game. The Hippocratic Oath is pretty well by the boards when it comes to welfare patients. Motivation for physicians is strictly financial." Dr. George Warner of the New York State Health Department echoed the same theme:

> I'm afraid our findings bear out the complaints of the nursing home people—that many and perhaps most attending physicians don't give their long term care patients adequate care. We find that they are relying too heavily upon tranquilizers and sedatives in the management of these people; that too often, they substitute a vague phrase such as 'senile' for a precise diagnosis which might lend itself to treatment; that their records and progress summaries for these patients are wholly inadequate.[2]

There is abundant evidence to support the proposition that the conduct of doctors who do visit nursing homes is far from exemplary. Daphne Krause, executive director of the Minneapolis Age and Opportunity Center, provided the following excerpts from sworn affidavits:

- From the affidavit of LPN Nancy L. Fox, re: The Kenwood Nursing Home (excerpt of a letter she sent to the doctor):

  Since you are the house doctor of the Kenwood Nursing Home, I have, for quite some time now, observed your approach to these elderly patients.

  Your last visit occurred a couple of weeks ago. On that day you arrived early and I had not yet put on my nurse's cap. The supervisor was off all day and you assumed, obviously, that I was an aide.

  All 13 patients had been psychologically prepared for your visit. I had told them you were coming and to be sure to explain all those things which had been bothering them...that you would listen and do all you could to relieve their anxiety and pain. They were all awaiting your visit with high hopes.

  Unknown to you, Doctor, I timed your visits with them. You started rounds at 9:50 a.m. You finished at 10:10 a.m. That meant that you spent exactly 1-1/2 minutes, on the average, with each patient. Not one of them did you examine. Your satchel remained on a chair in the hall, unopened. You handed out new orders as glibly as one scatters seed to the birds....

  One patient, in particular, you insulted. You said to... (him), when he complained legitimately of his chronic severe back and other pains: 'All you need to do... is to go out and find yourself a nice blonde.'... The patient can hardly walk and shakes violently nearly all the time.

- From the affidavit of nurse's aide Barbara Lace, re: the David Herman Nursing Home:

  At the home there are people who have not seen a doctor in 2 years. In the time I have been there, I think I have only seen a doctor three times. I don't see how a doctor can prescribe medications and treatment to a patient over the phone. This is done all the time.

- According to the affidavit of nurse's aide Gladys E. Danielson, re: the Bryn Mawr Nursing Home: A patient, Mrs. X, at the Bryn

Mawr Nursing Home was transferred to the nursing home after a bladder operation. The staff told the aides that the stitches should come out in two weeks.

I talked to the nurse administrator, Mrs. Coleman, and she said it would be taken care of Monday. Then on Monday I asked her if the stitches were to come out and she said, "No, let the doctor do it." So I let it go at that and continued to take care of her every morning. Then I was gone from work there until she died.

- From the affidavit of Gloria Johnson, the daughter of the patient just mentioned, re: the Bryn Mawr Nursing Home.

There was no follow-up by the doctors from Methodist Hospital, nor did Bryn Mawr see to it that her postsurgical condition was checked or her stitches removed by a doctor.... On May 12, 1970, my mother entered the Bryn Mawr Nursing Home. At no time from the point she left Methodist Hospital to the day she died on June 12, 1970, did she see a doctor.... I have since contacted the Minnesota State Board of Health to complain of the negligent treatment my mother received. I was informed by Mrs. Ruth Larson of the State Board that at no time did the Bryn Mawr Nursing Home even have any medical records of my mother. They did not even know what she had been operated on for at Methodist Hospital.

Numerous scientific studies have uncovered similar cases of negligence. For example, a 1971 study conducted by the Connecticut Department of Health was critical of physicians' record-keeping habits and inattention to patients. The report stated that it was impossible to tell if the patient was receiving care adequate to his needs. Another aspect of this study was the frightening conclusion that essential lab tests were not being completed on about 40 percent of all the nursing home patients in the sample. Moreover, almost 40 percent of patients taking cardiovascular drugs such as digitalis had not had their blood pressure taken in more than a year.

A similar study of 75 nursing homes in two cities was prepared in 1971 by Carl I. Flath, a consultant to the Health Services and Mental Health Administration, Department of Health, Education, and Welfare. It reports these startling results:

- More than 30% of the patients had no recorded admission data, no transfer abstract, no diagnosis, nor initial treatment orders — even though many of them already were on digitalis and other potentially dangerous drugs.
- 73% had no recorded admission history.
- 66% had not been given an admission physical examination; and of the physicals that were recorded, less than a third covered more than three of ten body systems.
- Only 30% had an admission urinalysis, and less than 30% had an admission hemoglobin/hematocrit.
- Only 13% had any long range medical or social planning recorded.
- 15% had no written diet orders.
- More than 50% of the patients had no weights recorded at any time during their stays.
- 25% of the patients taking heart medication such as digitalis had no diagnosis of heart disease on their charts; 33% of those taking insulin had no diagnosis of diabetes.

This data is confirmed by still other government reports. On July 15, 1974, Thomas Tierney, the director of the Bureau of Health Insurance transmitted to the Senate Finance Committee a status report on the more than 4,000 Medicare-participating nursing homes. The study showed that 2,068 homes were in violation of one or more of the physician's requirements:

- 374 homes were in violation of the requirement that telephone orders for patients received by the nursing homes must be countersigned by the physician within 24 hours.
- 340 homes had treatment orders in effect that were out of date (treatment orders can be prescribed for only 30 days) and some in effect for long periods of time, six months or a year.
- 288 homes did not conform to the standard requiring that a medical evaluation of the patient's needs be completed within 48 hours after admission.
- 217 homes failed to carry out the requirement that physicians make arrangements with fellow physicians to care for their patients in the facility in the event of the absence of the patient's primary physician.

Inadequate Drug Control

Chapter 3 details the lack of control on drugs and the generally haphazard method of distributing them in nursing homes. Physicians are at least partly to blame. Most medications are prescribed over the telephone. In fact, one administrator testified that if it wasn't for Alexander Graham Bell, there would be no medicine practiced in U.S. long term care homes.

There is no need at this point to repeat the dangers documented in Chapter 3 beyond the following quotation from a study by Dr. Bernard A. Strotsky and RN Joan R. Dominick, who underline the importance of close supervision of drugs by physicians:

> Patients who are on maintenance doses of medication for chronic conditions should be reevaluated regularly. Digitalis toxicity; diuretic-induced dehydration, weakness, hyperglycemia, hypokalemia and hypochloremia; and phenothiazine-induced Parkinsonism, hypotension, blood dyscrasias, dermatitis, and mood changes occur with alarming frequency in patients.[3]

Failure to Report Infectious Disease: The Baltimore Salmonella Epidemic

The most commonly accepted theory explaining the Baltimore salmonella epidemic is that on Sunday night, July 26, 1970, some 146 patients and some of the employees of the Gould Convalescent Center consumed a meal containing a virulent strain of salmonella bacteria. On Monday the home was confronted with a mass outbreak of diarrhea. More and more patients became ill on Tuesday and Wednesday. Some patients' physicians were called.

Some of the 44 physicians having patients in the facility came to visit them. The home's legally required "Principal Physician," Dr. Harold Harbold, responsible for the largest number of patients, was on vacation. The physicians who did visit the facility chose to claim responsibility for only their own patients. Not one doctor reported an infectious disease or in any way alerted the state to the possibility that it might have a major epidemic on its hands. By the time the state first learned of the outbreak on Friday, July 31, more than 20 patients had died. All in all, 36 patients died.

This tragedy focused attention on three facts which have been documented in other contexts as well.

- In most states, no one physician has the responsibility for the kind of medical care offered in a nursing home. Everybody and nobody is responsible. Titles such as "Medical Director" or "Principal

Physician" exist in law or regulations, but there are seldom more than paper requirements.

- Physicians in the U.S. are lax in reporting infectious diseases, and nursing homes need to give greater attention to the isolation of patients with such diseases.
- Physicians in the U.S. routinely sign death certificates of patients who have died in nursing homes without having viewed the body.

With respect to the first point, Senator Moss was successful in getting HEW to issue regulations to require all nursing homes participating in Medicare of Medicaid to have designated medical directors. However, whether or not this provision will be enforced by HEW remains to be seen.

As noted in Chapter 2, the hearings on the salmonella epidemic amply underscored the casual manner in which most physicians treat infectious diseases. Less than one percent of such diseases are reported each year. The penalties for not reporting are minor. Often, the fine is less than $100. Despite repeated warnings, few additional precautions have been taken. As a result, the elderly in nursing homes continue to be an extremely high risk population, and the possibility of another salmonella epidemic is very real.

Dr. Jesse Steinfeld, then surgeon general of the U.S., and Dr. David Sencer, director of the Communicable Disease Center in Atlanta, Georgia, both testified that the Maryland food poisoning experience could be repeated in any nursing home throughout the nation. They were unanimous in the need for more rapid reporting and more vigorous treatment for these diseases.

Death Certificates

The investigation of the facts of the Baltimore epidemic also revealed the fact that doctors commonly signed death certificates without seeing the bodies of patients who died in nursing homes and that there was no Maryland law requiring them to do so. These facts were disclosed by the General Accounting Office, which reported this to be the common practice across the country. In fact, GAO revealed that only two states have legal requirements requiring physicians to view bodies before signing death certificates, reporting: "It is not an uncommon practice for physicians to sign death certificates without first viewing the bodies. GAO interviewed physicians, most of whom felt it was 'either impractical or unnecessary to view bodies of patients who had died in nursing homes.' "

The folly of this practice was indicated by Dr. Jesse Baron, who has written:

> Some studies have shown that [the elderly] patients will die because the doctor will say the patients are too old to be operated upon. The death will be attributed to old-age diseases like arteriosclerosis but the autopsy will show it was diabetic coma or peptic ulcer — something which could have been treated.[4]

Dr. William J. Curran of Harvard University, an expert on legal medicine, makes the same point when arguing the need for better investigations of deaths. Dr. Curran reports that the U.S. regards death a bit more casually than European countries. He indicates an "urgent need" for more medico-legal investigations, particularly because of the increased use of drugs in American medicine. Given the loose control of drugs in U.S. nursing homes generally, there is ample reason to pay more attention to the causes of patients' deaths.

Dr. Frank Furstenburg, medical director of Mt. Sinai Hospital and the Hebrew Home and Infirmary, Baltimore, Maryland, agreed that it is advisable for doctors to view the bodies of patients who had died in nursing homes. He pointed out that there are proportionately a greater number of accidents and injuries in nursing homes which go unreported.

Conclusion

Except for the few who have made geriatrics their life's work, doctors avoid nursing homes. The consequences are clear. Patients go without the medical care they need. The RNs, LPNs and aides are deprived of the direction and supervision that they need. More than likely, their only contact with the physician is by telephone. The result is an intolerable burden on the few RNs who work in nursing homes. Ultimately, homes rely on the untrained and unlicensed aides and orderlies to provide needed care and services. The result is a virtual guarantee of poor care.

Chapter 13

Nursing Homes without Nurses

Nursing homes, as their name seemingly implies, might be expected to place major responsibility for patient care upon nurses. But the name is misleading. Within the context of a nursing home, the word "nurse" is used very loosely to apply to almost everyone in white. In reality, there are only about 65,000 registered nurses in today's 23,000 long term care facilities, who care for over a million patients. And this number must be divided by three: the morning, afternoon, and night shifts needed for 24-hour care.

The importance of RNs in nursing homes is obvious from previous references, but an even greater understanding of this role is essential. RNs must complete a minimum of two years of education at an accredited school of nursing. They should be thought of as the hub of the nursing home wheel. Ideally they should provide a great deal of direct nursing care. Indeed, there are certain nursing functions which only RNs are competent to perform. These include dressings of all kinds; clysis; catheter insertion and changes; impactions; tube feedings; oxygen therapy; Q/A intravenous, subcutaneous and intramuscular injections; dispensing medications; ostomy irrigations and care; urological irrigations; ear and eye irrigations; lavage and gavage; isolation; suctions; and assistance with thoracentesis and paracentesis.

As RNs will be quick to tell you, there are great risks involved if the above chores are performed by untrained personnel. They point out that nursing is a profession, and only through training and experience can appropriate judgments be made. The results of inadequate professional nursing care can be seen in many U.S. homes. One common example is patients with bedsores or contractures (stiffening of the muscles and joints).

But nurses perform other important tasks in nursing homes, and that is supervising the work of others. The task may include hiring and firing nursing personnel, in-service training, checking of housekeeping and dietary personnel, maintaining patients' records, consulting with physicians, administrators, and therapists, and serving on a host of committees such as the utilization review committee and the infection control committee.

From this quick analysis, it is easy to see that work in a nursing home is very demanding from an RN's point of view. But what other reasons explain the scarcity of nurses in nursing homes? The answer is complex, a conglomerate of many reasons.

Few Nurses Are Required by Law

Despite a major battle over the last ten years, nursing home interests have prevailed over the public interest and federal requirements, for the number of nurses remains low. In so-called skilled nursing homes, only one registered nurse is required on the day shift (7 a.m. to 3 p.m.), seven days a week. Only one licensed practical nurse (LPN) must be on duty on each of the afternoon and evening shifts, no matter what the size of the nursing home. The inadequacy of this standard can be seen by comparing it with various state standards. For example, Connecticut requires one RN for every 30 patients on the morning shift, one for every 45 patients on the afternoon shift and one for every 60 patients in the evening shift. Nursing home operators have continually opposed such minimum ratios even though they were contemplated (but never implemented by HEW) as part of the 1967 Moss amendments.

This obviously serious problem becomes even more so when one reflects that the second category of federally supported nursing homes, intermediate care facilities, are not required to have an RN on duty at any time. The basic standard calls for one LPN on duty eight hours a day, seven days a week. Pathetic and anemic as they are, even these minimum federal standards have never been enforced.

Poor Working Conditions

Other reasons for the absence of nurses are poor working conditions, lower wages and fringe benefits, and the image of nursing homes. Nurses, like doctors, to a greater extent than most, need a feeling of self-satisfaction. They need to feel that they are useful and effective and have contributed to the well-being of humanity. This sense of satisfaction is available in hospital work but is not thought to be available in a nursing home. Dr. Victor Kassel put it this way, "The nursing home is the low rung on the ladder. Nurses who have been in the hospital will not accept a job in a nursing home, even if you pay them a good salary. If they do take a job somebody will ask, 'Why are you in a nursing home; where did you foul up?'"

Mary E. Shaughnessy, RN, speaking for the American Nurses' Association, and Assistant Dean of Nursing Lois Knowles, of the University of Florida, stated there are really two sets of reasons, one obvious and the other hidden. Nurse Shaughnessy told the committee, they were:

(a) Nursing homes do have a poor image as far as nurses are concerned. (b) The average nurse is ill prepared to meet the needs of elderly people with long-term complex medical problems, without supplementary training. (c) The difficulties of practicing safe nursing care according to accepted standards of practice are very great due to the restricted policies or lack of policies in many of these institutions. (d) The lack of authority vested in the nursing service department makes it very difficult to carry out the kind of care that is required. (e) The isolation of the nursing home from other health facilities makes it an unpopular place to practice. (f) The lack of stimulation and support from other nurses, physicians, and other health workers is another factor. (g) The poor administration, overall administration of many of the facilities prevents well prepared nurses from continuing to work in them.

The Unclear Role of Nurses

The less obvious reasons that nurses avoid nursing homes has to do with the design of long term facilities and the delivery of services to their residents. Dean Knowles notes that a small hospital design has been followed. Mary Shaughnessy calls this the "dilution of the kind of services we have in hospitals by two-thirds or one-half." They conclude that little attention has been paid to clarifying and communicating the product nursing homes offer. The public, they claim, has only a hazy idea of what constitutes good nursing. What is needed, they assert, is a total rethinking of the needs of nursing home patients from the point of view of clinical geriatric nursing. Shaughnessy strongly suggests that in redefining nursing practice in long term care facilities, nurse practitioners trained in geriatrics might be one solution.

Few Nursing Schools Emphasize Geriatrics

Few of the 1,054 schools of nursing in the United States have emphasized geriatrics. This was the conclusion we reached after evaluating replies to a questionnaire sent to each school asking:

- Does your program now include or are you planning to make geriatrics a specialty in your curriculum?
- Do you have a program whereby students or interns can fulfill requirements by working in nursing homes?
- Does your nursing program in any other way service nursing homes?

Of the 512 returns received, only 27 answered the first question in the affirmative; 274 answered that geriatrics was included in their curriculum as part of a more general course on human development; and only 135 answered that they had a program whereby students worked with nursing homes.

Assuming that those who had programs in geriatrics would have been the most likely to return the questionnaire, the result confirms that comparatively few schools of nursing emphasize geriatrics to a significant degree. If additional proof were needed, it can be found in the April 1975 study, "Nursing and Long-Term Care: Toward Quality Care For the Aging," a report prepared by the American Nurses' Association for the Subcommittee on Long Term Care.

Few Government Programs Emphasize Geriatrics

By the most recent tally, there were 144 separate programs administered by 13 separate agencies for the training of nurses and health care personnel. Some 94 of these programs were exclusively for the training of nursing personnel and together received $1.7 billion in fiscal 1973. It is impossible to separate the portion of the other 50 programs that went for the training of nurses; thus, no one knows exactly how much money is being spent to help train nurses. But up until the present time there has been little utilization of these programs to train personnel specifically for nursing homes and little on geriatric nursing generally. In fact, according to the aforementioned ANA study, there are no graduate programs in gerontological nursing anywhere in the United States at the present time.

THE EFFECT OF THE SHORTAGE OF NURSES

Much has been written about the nurse shortage, with the Department of Labor reporting a shortage of about 150,000 nurses. As always, nursing homes are at the bottom of graduates' lists. A true shortage would explain the absence of nurses in nursing homes to some degree, but there are times when a shortage is not really a shortage. Dr. John Mason of the American Lutheran Church told the committee that good nursing homes have no difficulty attracting nurses, even in rural areas where they are in shortest supply.

Mary Shaughnessy, testifying for the American Nurses' Association, told the committee that there are about 400,000 RNs who have dropped out of the work force. Many have dropped out to have families, but a substantial number have dropped out for other reasons, such as "inadequate definitions of the nurses' role in the organization, poor communication and coordination and unreasonable work pressures." More and more, nurses are demanding a larger role in health care and no longer wish to see themselves as the "physician's technical assistant" or the "patient's servant."

Another reason for the "nurse shortage" is the commitment of RNs to administrative rather than nursing duties in U.S. nursing homes. The accumulated evidence indicates that the RN in a nursing home spends comparatively little time tending to patients. Time and motion studies conservatively indicate that nurses spend an alarming 54 percent of their time on non-nursing activities. These studies report that administrative and clerical work, such as ordering supplies, preparing forms, and answering telephones, consumed 40 percent of the RN's time. Other nursing tasks, many of which could be performed by nurse's aides (e.g., making beds and bathing patients), accounted for three percent of the nurse's time, and non-work activities such as socializing, reading non-nursing magazines, eating meals and attending to personal hygiene accounted for 14 percent. In short, only 43 percent of the time was spent on tasks properly performed by the registered nurse, such as administration and recording of medications, preparing nurse's notes and instructions, or supervising other nursing personnel.

In short, there are comparatively few RNs in nursing homes, and the ones who do work there are generally overworked and overburdened with administrative duties. The same can be said of the 45,000 licensed practical nurses who function in the stead of the RN. LPNs are in charge in the absence of the RN. They must perform the supervisory, care-giving, and administrative functions. The inevitable result is the reliance on unlicensed and untrained personnel to provide 80 to 90 percent of the care that is given in American nursing homes.

This is a rather startling statistic, but there is support for it from experts and from scientific studies as well as from common observation. For example, Dr. Raymond Benack, founder of the American Association of Nursing Home Physicians and president of the Maryland Association of Physicians in Chronic Disease Facilities, testified that 90 percent of the medical care in this country is being given by untrained and poorly educated aides and orderlies. Dr. Benack's view was supported by Mary Shaughnessy of ANÁ, David Mosher, former president of the American Nursing Home Association, and the Nader Task Force on Nursing Home Problems.

Firm support for this conclusion is also provided by an October 1970 HEW study which concluded that "Eighty-one percent of the nursing care tendered to patients was given by ancillary personnel." The report also comments that only seven percent of nursing home care was given by RNs. HEW admitted that the figure was somewhat lower than was expected, but explained, "The role of the RN in the nursing home is primarily one of administration and supervision of the nursing staff."

WHAT IS A NURSE'S AIDE?

In the words of a study by Len Gottesman of the Philadelphia Geriatrics Center, nurse's aides are responsible for bathing, dressing, toilet care, grooming, making beds, cleaning night stands, passing trays and fresh water, generally observing the well-being of the residents, conducting activities, shopping for residents, or setting and styling ladies' hair. Male nurse's aides who perform identical functions are called orderlies.[1]

Most nurse's aides and orderlies receive no training for their jobs; 53 percent of those applying have no previous experience. Aides have little formal education; only one-half of the 280,000 U.S. aides and orderlies are high school graduates. The turnover rate for aides is 75 percent a year. Some operators, then, argue that there is no use in training people who will stay only a few days and then move on. It is very easy to obtain a job as a nurse's aide or orderly in a nursing home, which may attract drug addicts and those with criminal records, because references are seldom checked.

The pay is low. Starting pay is usually the minimum wage of $2.30 an hour, or about $92 a week. Job benefits are typically few; days off are irregular and include only one or two weekends a month. Many aides report that they are often called and persuaded to work on their days off. Several have told us they would like a policy of providing aides with two consecutive days off.

The work is very hard and unpleasant. Few people relish employment calling for cleaning up after the abandoned members of society, many of whom are incontinent.

There is little hope for advancement. The chances for promotion are slim and wages will never get much beyond the minimum wage. As Dr. Gottesman wrote,

> It would be difficult to find in our society a working role more deserving of recognition and less recognized. We assign to this group of workers the role and the functions of family members. They give the care which relatives and friends are not available to give. We believe that most often they do it with gentleness and compassion. Yet we fail to define the role or develop it by means of even the most minimal requirements.

CONSEQUENCES OF RELYING ON UNTRAINED PERSONNEL

Virtually every major study of nursing home problems pinpoints the reliance on untrained personnel as a major cause of the poor care and abuse in nursing homes. Dr. Lionel Z. Cousin, clinical director of the United Oxford Hospital geriatrics unit in London, observed that the lack of sufficient numbers of professional nurses trained in geriatrics is the primary reason for our existing problems in the field of long term care. The Nader task force and Dr. Victor Kassel agreed. Dr. Charles Kramer, president of the Kramer Foundation and clinical director of the Plum Grove Nursing Home, told the committee:

> What I am trying to say is that most of the patient care is given by people with the least education in the psychology of people, the sociology of old age, and the dynamics of interpersonal relationships in the institution. This means that if you are going to give patients the kind of care they need, you have to train everyone in the institution.

Ida Mae Dentler, chairwoman of the Houston citizens' committee, HELP (Helpless Elderly Lonely People), after several years' investigation of Texas nursing homes, has arrived at the conclusion that 50 percent of the complaints against nursing homes in her state were caused by "unlicensed, uncontrolled health care workers." She has a long list of complaints compiled from her records, including drinking on the job, sleeping on duty, abusing patients, stealing their belongings, showering them in hot or cold water as punishment, eating their food, stealing medications, and intimidating senile patients by threatening to set them on fire.

Reporters Mike Richardson and Peggy Vlarebome of the *St. Petersburg Times*, working in many Pinellas County (Florida) nursing homes prior to writing a series on nursing home problems, were critical of the "learn-by-doing" method of training aides. They also provided this list of "Dos and Don'ts" accepted among many nurse's aides:

- Don't make trouble for your fellow employees. This means you don't report that the only nurse on the 3 p.m. to 11 p.m. shift is not licensed in Florida. "She is a good nurse," the 11 p.m. to 7 a.m. shift nurse tells you.
- Don't do anything you don't have to do. "The other shifts don't do any work, so why should we..."
- If you discover a wet bed at 2:30 a.m., don't change it until 5:30, "so we don't have to do it twice," a nurse advised.
- Don't use cups or utensils used by patients; "you don't know what you might get from them."
- Don't touch a runny bedsore because you might get a staph infection. Let the other shifts worry about the patients' getting staph infections.
- Don't waste your time talking to patients. "They're so senile they don't know what you're saying anyway."
- When you do talk to patients, talk as if they were children; don't ask if they have to go to the bathroom, ask, "Do you have to pee-pee?"
- Don't spend a lot of time feeding patients who can't feed themselves; they won't know the difference.
- If you have a headache, just ask the nurse for aspirin and she will give you some of a welfare patient's "and let someone else pay for it."
- Don't change the top sheet unless it is really soaked as the patient will be charged extra for it. Presumably the patient would rather be wet and get a urine burn.
- If patients "get in the way," strap and lock them in their chairs by day and their bed by night. Don't bother checking on them

"vigilantly" as required by State law — a law unknown to most caretakers and ignored by the others.
- If you have a patient who uses a catheter, "irrigate it when you get a chance" instead of every eight hours as required, a nurse said. Do it when you can — right or wrong.[2]

In his April 14, 1975 article on his investigation of nursing homes in Hawaii, *Honolulu Advertiser* reporter Harold Hostetler wrote, "The lack of proper staff is the root of most complaints about nursing home care in Hawaii. The problem is particularly acute in State-owned facilities, but all the homes share in the problem." He quotes a physician:

I think one of the biggest problems in nursing homes in Hawaii is the poor quality of floor help. There is a lack of supervision to look over the duties of the poor quality help which is poorly trained. It results in neglect — in patients lying in urine-soaked beds longer than necessary, and in rough handling of patients by the staff that don't have the training to understand what they are doing.

A DISPROPORTIONATE NUMBER OF AIDES ARE MEMBERS OF MINORITY GROUPS

A special and little-mentioned problem in this area is the fact that a disproportionate number of the nation's aides and orderlies are blacks or members of other minority groups. There are no firm statistics, but it is an educated guess that while minorities make up only four percent of nursing home patients, they probably make up about 25 percent of all nursing home aides.

This should not be too surprising in view of the fact that these people are most often paid the minimum wage and require no training as a prerequisite to employment. Large numbers of blacks and Mexican Americans who find it difficult to obtain jobs easily secure employment in nursing homes because of the industry's high vacancy and turnover rates.

In long term care facilities they find themselves taking care of a predominantly "Anglo" population. The best description of the interaction of these two groups is "The Current Social Revolution and Its Impact on Our Homes," a monograph by Herbert Shore, Ed.D., administrator of Golden Acres, Dallas, Texas, and former president of the American Association of Homes for the Aged. He says, in part:

Nursing care at the basic level is intimate, difficult, hard, dirty, and often unpleasant. The nurse's aide or orderly constantly faces fecal and urinary incontinence, bed sores, infection, reactions to physical discomfort and anguish of the patient and the physical agitation and insults of mentally disturbed or brain damaged patients. An uncomfortable or uncontrollable patient who lashes out angrily at a Black nurse and calls her "nigger," can't expect warm, tender loving care in return; nor should the family, although the institution does expect such positive approaches to care.

In large cities, very substantial majorities of nursing home and hospital employees, especially in the service and maintenance units, are made up of Black and other minority groups. What is the milieu from which the Black nurse's aide comes to start her work day? In the words of Mrs. Martin Luther King, Jr., the home or hospital employees of which we speak are 'sick and tired of being sick and tired'. She comes from and returns to substandard housing, overcrowded conditions, poor sanitation, and her inadequately cared for children, while she is away caring for others. She leaves a husband at home who may be underemployed or unemployed and who is overwhelmed with a sense of hopelessness and inadequacy.

Through their neighborhood action groups, union, and their news media, the Black or Mexican nurse's aide is constantly reminded that she is the victim of white exploitation and raw discrimination by the white power structure. This indoctrination amplifies and stereotypes for the Black home and hospital worker some of her own negative personal experiences.

These are the tensions that exist in her community and her orbit, and these are the hardened feelings with which she faces the day in attempting to provide physical care and emotional comfort to a very sick and sometimes hostile older patient. These are the persecutory and bitter feelings she must hold in check, while she powders the buttocks of an elderly and helpless patient whose bed may have to be changed several times a day due to fecal incontinence, or whose raw bed sores must be dressed with patience and care. This patient may be symbolic of all the misfortunes and indignities she has experienced. He is white and is surrounded by a solicitous family who may act toward the worker in a manner which appears patronizing and arrogant. The family reacts symbolically to the Black aide who in turn may respond with indifference or surliness. Without admitting to the prevalence of the situation described above, we cannot expect improvement in patient care.

In a related development, Daphne Krause discovered, and the Minnesota Health Department verified, an elaborate swindle to bring Korean girls into the United States on the pretense that they would receive formal training in a work-study arrangement. Korean girls were defrauded of about $700 prior to their departure for the United States. They had to pay their own airfare. Most of them could not speak or write English. Investigations revealed a complex and widespread problem with international implications. The girls were used routinely as aides in nursing homes. The facilities were taking advantage of an opportunity to gain cheap labor without attempting to provide the comprehensive training that the girls (and the Immigration Department) expected. The girls could not speak English and thus had difficulty in communicating with the patients. One promoter, who had advanced the airfare, secured agreements from nursing homes to subtract money from the wages paid the girls until the airfare was paid. One operator even withheld additional amounts from their minimum wage level salaries to cover the cost of room and board.

The aspiring Korean nursing students in this case did not have their visas renewed and had to return to Korea without the promised training. Evidence suggests that several hundred Korean girls entering the United States may have been duped in this manner.

Conclusion

Physicians are absent from the nursing home setting. Nurses are few and far between. The beleaguered nurses employed in nursing homes are grossly overworked and tied down with administrative duties and spend comparatively little time tending to their patients. The few licensed practical nurses who function in the stead of the RN as charge nurses in the other two shifts are also buried with paperwork and administrative duties. The result is that untrained aides and orderlies are providing 80 to 90 percent of the medical care in nursing homes.

The majority of these aides and orderlies have no training. They are paid the minimum wage for hard, unpleasant work. They have little or no hope for advancement and show a turnover rate of 75 percent a year. There is a distinct absence of any federal programs to provide in-service training for these individuals, whose training is pretty much trial and error. Some become competent, but most do not.

The end result is poor care. It was true in 1960 when the Subcommittee on Problems of the Aged and Aging issued its report on nursing homes. It is true today. A great number of the present nursing home abuses — perhaps as many as 50 percent — are directly attributable to this reliance on untrained and unlicensed personnel. All of these abuses have their roots in the fact that the least paid, the least trained, the least educated, and the least qualified members of the health care team have been given almost all of the responsibility for the forgotten one million elderly in U.S. nursing homes.

Part III
Positive Aspects in Long Term Care

The most recurrent and perhaps the most important questions in the field of long term care are: What makes a good nursing home? and How do I choose one? This section is an attempt to answer these questions for those shopping for a nursing home and to call attention to the fact that there are many fine homes in America.

Chapter 14
America's Finest Nursing Homes

[I] believe there is a growing and unfortunate trend to criticize all nursing homes under a blanket indictment. There are, and I want to emphasize, some very fine nursing homes across the country... at the same time there are serious problems. Our study and our preoccupation with these problems, I am afraid, sometimes adds to the impression that there is nothing positive in the nursing home field. I can categorically state that there has been great improvement in the past 10 years.

Senator Frank Church

TWO SCENES

In almost any American city there is one nursing home offering excellent care across the street from one offering poor care. What makes the difference? What makes a good nursing home? The following scenes may give some hint.

Scene I

When Frank Forester had his third stroke, it should have killed him; everyone said that—the doctor, his family, his friends—everyone. In fact, the stroke appeared to leave Frank more dead than alive. As months went by, the paralysis slowly left some parts of his body so that he had feeling in his right trunk and extremities. His right arm responded rustily, but his leg refused to answer his commands.

It was simply too much for his 80-year-old wife, with her failing health, to take care of Frank. Their only daughter lived half a nation away but flew in from time to time to help. Ultimately, they decided to place Frank in a nursing home. The local minister was consulted to recommend a good one near Frank's home. The clerk at the local welfare office was obliging, saying Frank's income was low enough to permit him to go in as a Medicaid patient.

One winter day, Frank was told that he was going to a nursing home where "things would be better" for his care. That same day his son-in-law helped move Frank and a few of his things into the institution. Nobody knew what Frank thought because his speech was still unintelligible.

At the nursing home Frank got lots of rest—just what he didn't need. No one came around to help him with his exercises. No one talked to him. He was sometimes helped out of his bed into a wheelchair and sometimes not, depending on whether Jenny came to work that day.

The fact that Frank was incontinent and that he was a welfare patient did not make him one of the home's favorites. He often spent hours in his own waste. Frank was supposed to take four different medications each day. Sometimes he got them and sometimes he didn't. Sometimes he got only two of his medications and occasionally he got the wrong medications—those intended for his roommate. When Frank became noisy (that is, attempted to communicate a complaint or a request for help), his reward was Thorazine or some other kind of tranquilizer, depending on which bottles were full in the medications room.

Nobody hurt Frank intentionally; nobody went out of the way to make life harder for him. Some aides were as kind as they could be, particularly Jenny. Others didn't have the time; they made their job kind of a race to see who could touch all the patients on their floor and return to the nurses station the fastest. For those who cared, there was much too much work to do. Little wonder the home often smelled of urine. Paradoxically, the linen closet and the closet with the toilet paper and supplies were kept locked, but anyone, even the untrained aides, had access to the medications room and the narcotics box. There was a definite shortage of mops and cleansers and maintenance men.

Frank watches a lot of TV, or seems to. No one knows for sure.

This scene does not date back to another decade or century. It is happening today in many of America's nursing homes.

Scene II

When Frank Forester entered this nursing home, his family was impressed by the continual activity. Standing in the central intersection of the home, they could see people in white uniforms helping patients walk, involving them in activities: inspiring them to live and rewarding them for performance.

The day Frank arrived they were having a birthday party for Mrs. Jackson, who had just turned 102. All the residents were there for cake. Frank's son-in-law thought the beer and wine were a nice addition to the party but commented that it was "pretty far out" for a nursing home.

Frank was given a physical by the home's medical director on Wednesday and saw the doctor again on Friday, the doctor's regular day at the home. The doctor and the registered nurse in charge set up a therapeutic program for Frank, along with his medication regimen designed to restore the movement he lost because of the stroke. Bright and early on Saturday morning, the RN talked to Frank about his program. She talked repetitively and slowly. On Sunday, Frank was wheeled to church services; after lunch the home had scheduled a movie — Douglas Fairbanks, Jr. in tight pants — and everyone enjoyed it.

After a few months of therapy, Frank gained greater use of his arm and began to talk a little. He began to enjoy his roommate's company as they talked about fishing and hunting. One Thursday after therapy, the home held senior citizens olympic games. Mrs. Flores won the beanbag toss at 75 feet. Frank placed third in men's frisbee at 50 feet. Two days later, all the home's residents, including those who were bedridden, were put into a customized schoolbus with a hydraulic lift and taken on a tour of the city. The patients enjoyed the Christmas lights, decorations, and hustle-bustle of people shopping. On the way home they encountered a fire engine enroute to a blaze. They followed in the bus and observed from a safe distance. Later, Frank enjoyed the visits from several groups of carolers even though his roommate grumbled each time they sang "Silent Night."

About 6 months later Frank was a much-improved man. Although he still had little control of his right leg, his speech was letter perfect; his thoughts were clear. One day that June, Frank enjoyed two memorable events in one day. He celebrated his 81st birthday — his wife and just about everyone was there. There were gifts and champagne. Then, in realization of his fondest wish, Frank got to go fishing. The home piled everyone who wanted to go into a bus and they went to a local pay-as-you-catch fishing hole. Frank caught six rainbow trout. As the fish were frying over the open picinc fire, Frank expressed gratitude to the administrator of the nursing home for making his life worth living.

This scene is not a look into the future. It too is happening today. What can be done to make this happy series of events more common in American nursing homes?

WHAT MAKES A GOOD NURSING HOME?

The subcommittee devoted considerable time to this question in view of its obvious importance. From the testimony of experts and hundreds of statements presented, it concluded, with Dr. James Folsom, the originator of "reality therapy," that the most important factor is a firm belief that the physical and mental problems of the elderly are, to a substantial degree, preventable and that even when these problems are present, they are more often than not reversible.

Dr. Muriel Oberlieder and most other experts agree that the second most important factor is a belief in basic human dignity expressed toward nursing home patients, not in the sense of doing everything for them, which makes them increasingly dependent, but in the sense of helping patients help themselves.

Witnesses before the subcommittee said again and again that good nursing homes are a matter of motivation. Of paramount importance to the quality of care is the administrator's ability to inspire his staff, to create the kind of harmony, unity of purpose, and spirit which makes a great symphony orchestra or which enabled the Green Bay Packers under Vince Lombardi to retain the world football championship year after year. Undoubtedly, there are many obstacles, but the fact that some administrators have succeeded so well against the existing odds is strong argument that others can and should follow suit.

In his appearance before the subcommittee, Dr. Karl Menninger underscored the importance of "team spirit," pointing out that rehabilitation is possible even for the aged with severe mental disabilities. Reading from his book, *The Vital Balance*, he described 88 patients in the geriatric ward of a Kansas mental hospital and what happened to them:

> They were not just old people. They were "crazy" old people. They were people whose relatives could not stand them, or did not want to stand them, or keep them. They were all dreary, dilapidated, hopeless people, waiting to die. Speaking rarely, spoken to rarely. Fifty-nine of these people were bedridden. About a score of them had no control over their excretory functions. They soiled the beds regularly. Forty-one of them were spoon fed at every meal. One of them had

been on the ward for 58 years. The average stay of these old people on this ward was 10 years!

Dr. Menninger went on to tell of how a young doctor and his staff transformed the hospital and of the immediate change in patients:

Each patient became a focus of attention. The ward was transformed from being a museum of dying human specimens into a hospital home in the best sense. Music and television were brought in. Cages of canaries, potted plants, aquariums were placed around the dreary halls, new lighting fixtures, drapes were installed, some of them by volunteers.

Birthday parties were held for each individual, and relatives were urged to come to these for weekend visits. A score of social activities were instituted with the combined aid of the patients, staff members, and volunteers.

The patients themselves painted a shuffleboard court on the floor of the previously sacred sitting hall. A ramp was constructed by the patients, over a short, but difficult flight of steps, which enabled some of the bed patients to be moved into the social center. Finger painting, furniture sanding, leather-tooling, bingo games, water-color painting, and all sorts of things were introduced.

A change in the clinical status of the patients was perceptible immediately. Three weeks after the program had begun, one patient was discharged to cooperative and interested relatives who were delighted to have their old father rise, as it were, from the grave and return to them.

By the end of the year only nine of these nearly 90 patients were still bedfast, and only six of them were still incontinent. Five had died. Twelve had gone home to live with their families. Six had gone out to live by themselves, and four had found comfortable nursing home provisions. Four of the original 88 were gainfully employed and self-supporting.[1]

Dr. Menninger commented that if this kind of improvement is possible with the most hopeless members in our society, then we should have high expectations for the rehabilitation of most nursing home patients.

The lesson appears to be that it is an intangible—esprit de corps—a sense of motivation manifested in individualized treatment and maximizing human dignity that marks the best nursing homes. Neither this esprit nor Tender Loving Care can be imposed by government fiat. It must be the result of the desire and commitment on the part of nursing home personnel. All American homes can provide superior care. All that is required is the *will* to do so.

WHAT PROGRAMS BEST SERVE TO REHABILITATE PATIENTS?

The principles and requirements of a good nursing home are well known to St. Joseph's Manor in Trumbull, Connecticut and Golden Acres in Dallas, Texas. At Golden Acres the team spirit concept is expressed as the LIFE program (Love, Interest, Fulfillment, and Enrichment). Personnel at Golden Acres and St. Joseph's Manor begin with the premise that every disabled adult can be rehabilitated. It is assumed that much lost function can be restored. The Crystal Springs Rehabilitation Center in San Mateo County, California also dedicates each and every staff member to this same goal.

In these facilities and other good homes, a variety of techniques have been developed which help upgrade the functional status of mentally impaired elderly patients. The techniques may be used singularly or in combination to modify unacceptable behavior and allow the patient's integration into a social group. Among these techniques are reality orientation, sensory training, and remotivation.

Reality orientation is a term for a program developed by Dr. James Folsom whose basic aim is to put a regressed patient into renewed contact with the world around him. It can be conducted in a class or through informal interaction. Orientation is taken at its most basic meaning. If patients do not know their own names, they are taught. If they don't know where they are from, this is taught next. Then they are taught the day, week, month, and the year, their age, etc. Typically, patients may exhibit confusion for many weeks but once they are able to grasp any bit of information such as their names, the names of their spouses, their birthdays, etc., they begin to recall and to be able to use ever-increasing amounts of material previously known.

Sensory training is a program aimed at combatting the almost total dependence and the separation from life created by living in the totally protected environment of a nursing home. When patients sit in institutions staring into space, receiving total care, with nothing to do but breathe, swallow, and excrete, dependence develops to the point where they no longer care about present realities. Sensory training supplements basic reality orientation by stimulating the patient's sensory sensitivity. As implemented at the White Plains Center for Nursing Care, patients are gathered together in small groups and asked to identify objects by smell, taste, hearing, touch, and sight. The program is useful for patients who manifest psychomotor retardation and poor discrimination between and response to environmental stimuli. Dr. Michael B. Miller, medical director of the facility, claims the program demonstrated that even severely brain-damaged patients can, with social encouragement and the warmth and affection of a compassionate leader, respond with increased feeling, increased thought, and even increased coordination. He echoes the message of Drs. Folsom and Oberlieder, "We know that senility need not be a fixed condition. There is much that is reversible about brain syndrome and senility." Dr. Miller continues that rehabilitation is doomed to failure unless it considers the whole person, adding psychological and social therapy to medical techniques.

Remotivation is a technique which was developed in the mental hospital some years ago. Essentially, it is an effort to find out what activities the patient enjoyed doing in earlier life, or would have liked to do, and directing him to those same goals. It can involve the use of rewards of many different types. Allowing a patient to participate in activities he enjoys is one form of reward. Certain foods or candy can be given as a reward along with the verbal "feedback" and reinforcement for increased effort and motivation.

Dr. Salvatore P. Lucia, professor emeritus of preventive medicine at the University of California, is the leading advocate of the judicious use of wine in nursing homes as a gentle non-toxic tranquilizing agent. Dr. William Dock of the Veterans Administration Hospital in New York agrees that wine has much to offer in the context of nursing home therapy. Dr. Robert Kastenbaum, professor of psychology at Wayne State University, also describes wine as beneficial. In addition to its use as a reward for increased function and independence or as a gentle tranquilizer, it is contended that wine has important psychological effects, making patients more socially oriented. Wine also supplies needed vitamins and minerals as well as being a "ready energy" food which requires minimum metabolic effort on the part of the body. Wine also stimulates the appetite and increases the flow of digestive juices, functions often slowed down in old age. From Dr. Kastenbaum's study, patients taking a glass of wine at night slept better with more "delta sleep" (deep refreshing sleep) than patients taking sleep-inducing sedatives. In addition, there are few contraindications in the use of wine, particularly in cooking where wine does much to enhance the flavor of food. For these reasons, more and more nursing homes are looking to the use of moderate amounts of wine for their patient population—subject always to physician's approval.

WHAT IMPROVEMENTS CAN BE MADE IN NURSING HOME DESIGN?

The physical structure of a nursing home has far-reaching effects on the quality of care and on the attitudes of its resident population. A few suggestions for the use of design to improve nursing homes follow: (1) As far as is possible within existing building codes, avoid the institutional appearance. Many modern nursing homes present a totally antiseptic environment. One witness told the subcommittee that nursing homes have been made so germ free and sterile that "human beings can't live there either." (2) Capture all the natural light you can. The use of skylights, ample windows and glass sliding doors can do much to eliminate that "closed in feeling." (3) Don't be stingy with common areas. A huge central fireplace or a solarium can soon become a favorite place for residents to congregate. The attraction of such a cozy nook may help motivate some withdrawn or reluctant patients to leave their rooms and participate in group activity. (4) Take advantage of nature. Most of us like to get out into the open air, to catch a little sun or just to get closer to nature. An open central court or a fenced-in back yard with abundant trees and flowers (and maybe even some animal life) would be a joy to many patients. (5) Individualize patients' rooms and their areas within their rooms. This allows them some sense of "territory"—a primal need. It allows them to feel unique and different from their neighbors. (6) Consider the advantages of a star-shaped design, or a floor plan in the pattern of an "X". These designs permit home personnel to stand in the center of the facility and have immediate line of sight throughout the entire structure. (7) Consider the advantages of saw-toothed walls in patients' rooms, but allow no more than two beds per room. In the saw-toothed concept, patients' rooms jut out at right angles for the entire length of the facility. This permits all patients (two to a room) to have their own windows. Moreover, it allows patients' beds to be placed at right angles, head to foot; thus, communication is easier and there is no coughing in the other patient's face as there would be if the beds were parallel. The location of the beds also makes it easy for the nursing staff; both patients can be seen at a glance just by opening the door. (8) Consider the virtues of individual thermostats for heat or air conditioning and a private sink, toilet, and shower in every room. These conveniences can do much to add to the patient's sense of comfort and dignity. (9) Make good use of color. Avoid drab institutional colors. Bright happy colors increase the likelihood that residents will enjoy their rooms. Appropriate use of color can also help keep patients from stumbling into furniture. The furniture should contrast with the walls and floors.

Painting doors different colors can help distinguish a closet from a hall or bathroom. Light switches can be more identifiable with color or luminiscence. Use of colors in corridors helps patients get about more easily. You may want to paint a colored stripe on the floor, a foot or more from the wall, which will help the elderly judge distance or serve as a guide for a wheelchair or walker. Handrails are more obvious if they are brightly painted. You may want to consider notching them to differentiate one hall from another. (10) Consider the use of carpeting on the floors. Even though it stains and in the long run is more costly to keep up than tile, carpeting adds warmth. It is also easier on the feet of both employees and patients.

WHAT IMPROVEMENTS CAN BE MADE IN EMPLOYEE TRAINING?

The training of nursing home employees, particularly aides and orderlies, is an important and difficult task. Many nursing homes have started excellent programs for this purpose. Ironically, once employees are trained, they quite often move on to work in hospitals where the pay is better and the work less arduous. The extent of this problem can be seen in the turnover rate of 75 percent a year common to such employees. While some nursing home operators have become cynical, the majority still realize the importance of these training programs. Following are a few examples of programs that have been organized. They are very much a "bootstraps" operation because, unfortunately, there is precious little federal money available for this purpose.

Accident Prevention Programs

Many nursing homes reported establishing accident prevention programs aimed at minimizing the possibility of injury or accident to patients or to the staff. Such programs have taken on new importance in view of the Occupational Health and Safety Act, which requires each employer to provide his employees with a safe place to work.

In-Service Training Programs

The Fredrick D. Zeman Center for Instruction in New York City is one of the best offering such programs. Under the direction of Dr. Manuel Rodstein, the center has an enrollment of 200 volunteers, doctors, and administrators. The cost of a standard course is $35, which covers a wide variety of topics from death and dying to institutional housekeeping and laundry management.

Another unique approach to in-service education is the Mobile In-Service Training to Nursing Homes in Phoenix, Arizona. The project is coordinated through the Phoenix Community College. The mobile unit's prime purpose is to update training for professional and allied health personnel and to promote better coordination of patient care in nursing homes, extended care facilities, and home health services. Contracts are signed by the institutions using the service, specifying the hours of training and the programs desired. The facility is charged $15 for each hour the unit is actually in the facility.

The mobile unit provides direct teaching in formal and informal classes, and at the bedside. In addition, it utilizes closed circuit FM radio broadcasts from the college district radio station. The variety of programs offered is remarkable: from 20-hour geriatric nursing assistant classes to much briefer staff in-service training in nursing audit and crisis intervention.

Continuing Education Programs

Continuing education programs are usually lengthier and more formal than in-facility, in-service education, and are focused on an area of concern rather than a specific problem. Continuing education may be offered by a long term care facility for their employees and outside individuals. For example, the Jewish Home and Hospital for the Aged in New York City conducts the following courses and workshops relating to care of the elderly:

Activities leadership
Nursing home administration
Behavioral sciences
Institutional management
Management and leadership
Geriatric medicine
Geriatric nursing
Nutrition for the geriatric patient
Occupational therapy
Physical therapy
Psychiatry and neurology of the aged
Remotivation
Residents' councils
Sensory deprivation
Social services

Many nursing homes have established mutually beneficial relationships with schools of nursing. For example, the Swope Ridge Nursing Home in Kansas City, Missouri is affiliated with Avilla College, as well as with several other schools of nursing in the Kansas City area. Students spend several days each semester in the facility observing the care of the chronically and mentally ill elderly. Moreover, the Missouri Division of Employment, which administers the manpower training program for licensed practical nurses, sends LPNs to Swope Ridge for clinical experience.

Training Senior Citizens to Work in Nursing Homes

The Senior Talent Opportunity Program (STOP) located in Minneapolis, Minnesota offers able-bodied senior citizens a three-week training course and pays them about $2.00 an hour while they train. When the course is completed, they join the staff of various area nursing homes at regular wages. This unique training program emphasizes good nutrition in health and illness, menu planning, food services, the psychological meaning of food and diet, and the feeding of stroke patients. This successful program may serve as the model for a wider, national program to train able-bodied seniors to work in long term care facilities.

Sensitivity Training

Perhaps the most impressive of the innovations the subcommittee received with respect to the training of nursing home personnel was the program of sensitivity training in effect at the Beaumont Convalescent Hospital at Beaumont, California. Marshal Horseman, administrator of the facility, told the subcommittee that he requires each prospective employee in the facility to assume the role of a patient for 24 hours before employment. He feels this experience gives employees valuable perspective. Employees are groomed by their fellow employees, given baths, fed, wheeled about in hospital-type gowns that open in the back. They are put to bed early, at 8 or 9 o'clock, like the other nursing home patients, and are required to stay in bed, perhaps developing an understanding of how it feels to try to sleep with nurses out in the hall making noise and conversing while socializing or in the performance of their duties. Mr. Horseman contends there is nothing like being at the mercy of the staff, wheeled about in a hospital gown with its attendant problems of maintaining modesty and dignity to help a nurse's aide learn the lesson that nursing home patients are human beings with dignity rather than objects incidental to employment.

Institutional Councils

Yet another unique training program deserves mentioning. The Lutheran Home of Moorestown, New Jersey has established an institutional council. The council includes representatives from each shift and from every class of nursing home employees: RNs, LPNs, aides, kitchen and maintenance workers, as well as administrative personnel.

In short, the elected representatives of the home's staff set the policy for the home. By giving all employees a voice in the operation of the facility, petty grievances and complaints are quickly resolved. The result is a smoother running operation with less turnover.

WHAT KINDS OF ACTIVITY PROGRAMS DO GOOD HOMES OFFER?

A recent ad for color television sets in a leading nursing home journal describes TV as "therapy for patients on the mend." Color TV is also touted as therapy for the staff: "Helps stamp out nuisance calls from patients who just want someone to talk to," and therapy for the administrator: "Brings in added income without capital investment".

Fortunately, fewer and fewer nursing homes are falling for this ad. There is more and more emphasis in today's nursing homes on activity and recreational programs. Such programs can run the gamut from bingo to participation in residents' councils (self-government by nursing home patients).

Ethel Hudson, then director of restorative activities, Shoshone County Nursing Home, Silverton, Idaho, provided the subcommittee with a graphic example of the importance of such activity programs. She asserts that much more than entertainment is involved. Activities provide the means of interesting patients in their care; they motivate the patients to make improvements on a wide scale from functional ability to physical appearance. She testified:

> The philosophy of patient care at our nursing home is simply this—the total care of our patients is the only reason for our existence. Total care of patients includes all efforts to provide an environment which contributes to the mental, physical, emotional, and social restoration of the patient to a normal dignified individual. Every effort of each member of our staff must be aimed to this end.

She noted that there were few activities when she took over her position in the home. "Our patients had little to look forward to except eating, sleeping and dying." One year after the activities program was instituted, the results were most encouraging. Bingo and movies were scheduled once a week, two one-hour craft classes were underway, and participation increased from five to about 40 patients.

One "heavy care patient," a chronic arthritic, produced a four-act play depicting the birth of Christ. The actors, directors, and stagehands were patients. The play had been slated for one performance, but its run was extended by popular demand. Four performances were given to more than 600 patients, staff, and members of the public. She described other activities the home offered, including:

Fishing, fly-tying, cabinetmaking, and furniture repair and finishing by one of our patients, a paraplegic; huckleberry picking, winemaking and to-scale dollhouse making by another of our patients, a double amputee.... Maintenance of a patriotic flower garden which keeps four of our patients busy during this season ....

We have recently installed a chapel for use by all denominations. Aside from worship services, this chapel is used for prayer and meditation, as well as an area for patient-family-minister solace and conferences. The finished decoration and the drapes for the chapel will be completed by the patients.

We hope soon to acquire and install a six-leather-pocket pool table for the use of our men patients. Each week at a scheduled period we have a session of card playing for men only. At these sessions the men patients play poker, pinochle, cribbage, and so forth, for 2 hours. Although money is not involved, chips are used for example in poker. The one who finishes with the most chips, the highest score, or runs the cribbage board most, wins a six pack of beer to take to his room to consume at his leisure, with his physician's permission.

She went on to describe cocktail parties, picnics, birthday parties, and dances staged by the patients themselves. Local civic groups paid for the musicians and some of the refreshments. "These activities added social confidence to our patients, and brought back many of their earlier, pleasant memories. This in turn, whets their memory recall, thus enhancing their mental alertness."

Ethel Hudson had the facts to prove her contention. Well over two-thirds (67 patients) of the patients admitted to the nursing home were classified as "heavy care" at the time of their admission. Largely because of the operation of the activities program, the number of patients so classified a year later was reduced to 9. She summed up:

> Our patients, who average 81.9 years of age, have taken a new outlook on life. The rather heavy Restorative Activities schedule, which is geared to patient interests and demands, gives our patients little time for idleness or for worrying about their condition or their problems. Due to a natural fatigue resulting from this active schedule our patients are, for the most part, sleeping naturally and without use of sleep-inducing medications.

Senior Citizens Olympics

A novel idea implemented a few years ago at the River Hills Nursing Home in Milwaukee, Wisconsin, in honor of the 1968 Olympic Games, was a Senior Citizens Olympic Games. Residents participated in shot put, discus, basketball throw, darts, javelin, shuffleboard, bowling on the green, skittle bowling, table bowling, and bean bag toss. Winners in individual events in each division, men and women, and in the decathlon received Olympic shields for first, second, and third place. It was reported that the idea was extremely well received even by those seniors who could only watch. The exercise was beneficial and the competition therapeutic.

Residents' Councils

There is a growing trend among nursing homes to establish residents' councils. Two states, New York and Wisconsin, were among the first to start this practice of self-government for nursing home patients. Some homes even allow the participation of members of the community on such residents' councils.

Consumer participation can only have positive results. At the very least, the program serves as a means of communicating to the home's administration problems which would not ordinarily come to their attention.

Dr. Florence Kavaler, former acting commissioner of the health and insurance program, New York City Department of Health, described such council meetings as a hybrid blending of town meeting, sensitivity session, pep rally, and forum. She says that communication is not just between the patients and the administrative and nursing staff;

there is communication among the residents. Both an educational and a recreational function are served.

She described one instance in which an aide had begun the practice of giving large numbers of patients their baths on the same morning, in assembly line "car wash fashion." At the residents' council meeting one patient complained about this practice, saying it was undignified. Others agreed and the astonished nursing home operator corrected the situation immediately.

Activities at the Iowa Soldiers' Home

No single activity or innovation can do the entire job that must be done in long term care. A total effort is needed on a variety of fronts. One of the most comprehensive efforts that reached the subcommittee's attention was that of the Iowa Soldiers' Home in Marshalltown, Iowa. There, staff must deal with the needs of domiciliary patients, others requiring skilled nursing, and still others needing more intensive care. In a letter, the administrator gave this list of efforts that might be regarded as "extras" in other facilities:

• Because many of the residents are handicapped and in wheelchairs, the grounds are planned for navigation by them.
• Tables are designed to have wheelchairs fit around them and ramps are provided as an alternative to stairs.
• The grounds feature several birdhouses for birdwatching residents.
• The little league baseball team plays on the grounds in summer.
• The home's grounds is the site of the annual community Easter egg hunt. Residents participate in hiding the eggs.
• Band concerts are held on the grounds through the courtesy of the local musicians union.
• The hills are used for sledding in winter, for parties and picnics in summer.
• Shuffleboard tournaments are held.
• Students working on degrees in nursing work with the residents in both degree and practical nursing programs.
• Reality orientation is practiced with calendars, clocks, and with signs over the patient's beds indicating name, home, and activities for the day.
• A program of government by patients is being tried with suggestion boxes available and meetings arranged between the administrator and the patients.

- There are no restrictions on visits; in fact, children are encouraged —a toy box is provided for their use.
- A rehabilitation kitchen is provided with all appliances adapted for use by the handicapped, including low sinks, radar ovens, and other kitchen aids. The elderly and handicapped can try their hand at preparing their own meals and can even participate in the shopping for these meals—in making lists and going to buy food.
- A library is provided with specially-designed furniture.
- There is a snack kitchen.
- Residents participate in small appliance repairing, wheelchair repair, woodwork, leatherwork, sewing, and quilting.
- A foreign food fair is held with residents dressing in the costumes of the country where their food originated and food is sold by "the taste."
- A fashion show is held with residents participating; likewise, there is a wig show and a hat show.
- Periodically one of the local department stores brings goods and opens a branch in the nursing home for a short while to enable the residents to buy a few needed items.
- Visits are arranged for Miss Iowa and Miss U.S.A.
- Residents prepare Christmas cards to send to families and friends.
- Costume parties are held with prizes.
- Bulletin boards commemorate birthdays with photographs of residents as well as charting the daily activities.
- Adult education is provided in painting, secretarial work, dancing, welding, typing, and biblical history.
- The home runs a toy repair service turning restored toys over to the Salvation Army for distribution.
- The home runs a Santa Claus answering service so that young boys and girls can call or write to the home and hear from Santa.
- A supper club activity is held monthly for residents who have little opportunity to eat in restaurants.
- Church services are provided for all denominations.
- The residents choose an employee of the month who receives a $25 savings bond.

Additional Activities at Other Homes

If all of the foregoing were not enough, following is a list of activities offered at various nursing homes: acting companies formed by residents, art shows and contests, barbeques, basketball from wheelchairs, bazaars, birthday parties, bingo, bridge, bar (alcoholic beverages served with consent of physicians), casino, cards, camping, ceramics, chinchilla raising, closed circuit television broadcasting, creative drama, croquet, dance therapy, dinner parties (each resident may invite two guests), dominos, exercise programs, fishing, gift shop for items made by residents, gardening, glee club, guest speakers, handicrafts, knitting, movies, music appreciation, newspaper publishing with extra large print, picnics, poker, parcheesi, pancake breakfasts cooked by residents, musical recitals, trips by bus to nearby areas of interest, travelogues, swimming, scrabble.

HOW CAN NURSING HOMES AID THE COMMUNITY?

More and more nursing homes are coming to understand that they no longer can survive as entities isolated from the mainstream of society. Isolation breeds suspicion and distrust. Accordingly, nursing homes are turning to community service, and by so doing are beginning to inspire public confidence.

Nursing homes that want to develop a positive image with their neighbors might consider the following: (1) Buy from local vendors. (2) Sponsor a Little League Baseball team. (3) Sponsor scholarships to help aspiring students, especially those intent on a career in nursing or medicine. (4) Contribute generously to bazaars and county fairs. (5) Sponsor programs to keep patients out of nursing homes. For example, provide foodstuffs for a local meals-on-wheels program or offer the use of your kitchen for the preparation of some of the meals. (6) Do everything you can to attract volunteers to help out in your home. Encourage them to form an advisory counsel. Be ready to accept their advice. (7) Do everything you can to encourage visits to your facility. Invite the mayor and local politicians to special ceremonies on holidays. Invite the press as well. (8) Join senior citizen representatives in lobbying for increased Social Security and other benefits for older Americans. Work hard for the elderly and earn their respect. (9) Sponsor a free day care program. Take care of children while their parents work. You may even want to offer free day care for aged adults. The cost will be minimal since you already have the facilities, and the benefits in good will will be well worth any minor losses or inconvenience you suffer. (10) Start an Adopt a Grandparent Program.

Patrick Norman, a medical student at the University of South Dakota at Vermillion, began the first such program in conjunction with the Dakota Nursing Home. In his program, college students entertain nursing home patients every Tuesday night with songs, skits, jokes, and cartoons. By last report, almost 100 students were participating in either the weekly entertainment or were making more frequent visits. About half of these students have "adopted" a grandparent.

One account of the program's success concerns a patient who was sent to the hospital with a coronary. She insisted that she be back at the nursing home on Tuesday, the night the "kids" come to visit. Physicians believe that this incentive was the reason for her speedy recovery.

The students are just as enthusiastic about the program, pointing out that they learned a great deal about life from their adopted grandparents. Outside observers confirm that the program is mutually beneficial. Some students have learned to crochet, one helped his grandfather build a birdhouse, and another baked a special pie for his diabetic grandmother.

The "Adopt a Grandparent Program" has reportedly been spreading throughout South Dakota to other colleges and even to some elementary schools. It has also been instituted at the Three Sisters Nursing Home in Indianapolis, Indiana with equally positive results.

Summing up, Ellsworth Cabot, director of The Chastian Homes, Inc., in Iowa, said that involving the nursing home and its personnel in the affairs of the community pays off in many ways. "Clergymen become frequent visitors," he says, "even doctors come with regularity and the local tax assessor is not likely to overassess a nursing home for which he has high regard."

HOW CAN INDIVIDUALS HELP NURSING HOME PATIENTS?

Following is a list of things that members of the community can do to aid nursing homes and nursing home patients. If we all would do our part, the all-too-common nursing home abuses would soon become only a faint memory of a distant past.

(1) Cooperate with local and national political leaders to establish participation of the elderly population in political action programs. The Gray Panthers are organized for just such a purpose. Nursing home patients, like all other citizens, have a right to vote and to influence the direction of the country. Many are not using their franchise at present. (2) Drive a nursing home patient to church. (3) Volunteer to set the hair for a patient or two. Pride in appearance does much to restore one's dignity and desire to go on living. (4) Teach a craft. (5) Help repair clothing. (6) Write and mail letters. Many patients have hands crippled with arthritis. (7) Take newspapers and magazines. Even trade papers will be of interest to some patients, reflecting news of a previous oc-

cupation. (8) Businesspeople can bring their merchandise to the elderly, as few can get to the store to buy needed clothes, tobacco, or other supplies. (9) Read to nursing home patients and establish one-to-one relationships with those having no family. (10) Organize or conduct various field trips for the elderly, in cooperation with the nursing home administrator. (11) Assist in feeding patients at meal time. (12) Correspond when you are away from the site or the facility. (13) Assist in handling personal affairs or run errands. (14) Share your babies with them—the sight of a newborn infant fascinates many oldsters. (15) Organize or participate with local organizations in watchdog "ombudsman programs" to oversee nursing homes. Community interest in nursing home patients is the best protection against substandard nursing homes. (See Appendix C for a list of such community action groups.) (16) Upon finding good care and services, write and spread the news. Write to your government representatives and newspaper to commend the administrator. Likewise, in finding abuses or poor care in your visits, write to your representatives and your local newspaper.

Chapter 15

How to Choose a Nursing Home

Perhaps three million families every year face the difficult decision of selecting a nursing home. Because a stay in a nursing home may continue several years, costing several hundreds of dollars a month, the purchase may be one of the most expensive you or your loved ones ever make. Few people realize *how* expensive. Projecting an average stay of 2.4 years and an average cost of $800 a month yields $22,400 as the cost of an average stay in a long term care facility. Even with so much money involved — to say nothing of the health, well-being and happiness of the patient — most people put little thought into the choice of a nursing home.

Most people look upon selecting a nursing home as unpleasant and postpone it until the critical day arrives. Under these circumstances, they are at a great disadvantage in negotiating with nursing home operators. It becomes very much a seller's market with the administrator in the position to say to a family desperately in need of assistance, "Take it or leave it." Families commonly accept the first available bed on terms dictated by a standard form contract which gives bountiful rights to the home (often including the right of summary eviction) and few to the patient. The tragedy of this situation is that patients are often placed in substandard or inappropriate facilities which a little research would reveal were less than adequate to meet their needs.

When Does a Person Need a Nursing Home?

People who need help dressing, who are incontinent, who cannot prepare their own meals, or who need some supervision so they will not bring harm to themselves are potential candidates for a nursing home. But before placing a person in a nursing home, families should check the availability of in-home services in their communities and the possibility that the patient's needs can be met short of institutionalization. More and more communities now have Home Health Agencies or Visiting Nurse Agencies which provide such in-home services including nursing care, physical therapy, or the services of a home health aide to help the elderly with their daily chores. In limited situations, the federal health care program for the aged, Medicare, or the program for indigents, Medicaid, may pay for some home health care. You should check this possibility, but do not expect too much since expenditures for in-home services constituted only about one percent of either program last year.

In the final analysis, only family members with the help of their physicians can judge when an individual's needs are both so intense and so unmet that placement in a nursing home is necessary. Most studies indicate that families do not readily abandon their elderly to nursing homes but do so only as a last resort.

WHAT KIND OF CARE DOES THE PATIENT NEED?

Many families are confused by the fact that nursing homes go by so many different names, including long term care facility, extended care facility, chronic disease hospital, convalariums, and shelter care facilities. Unfortunately, these labels and others seldom identify the level of care provided by the facility. There are really only two levels of nursing home care which take their names from the facilities that provide them. A skilled nursing facility (SNF) provides skilled nursing care; an intermediate care facility (ICF) provides intermediate care.

So that the reader may better understand these concepts, it may be helpful to see where these institutions fit into the spectrum of health care institutions. Most people are familiar with boarding homes (also called adult homes, domiciliary care facilities, etc.), which offer only board and room. One step above this are ICFs, which offer some nursing assistance and day-to-day supervision of patients. SNFs are the next step up. They offer intensive medical and nursing care including the 24-hour availability of licensed nursing personnel. The final step in the spectrum is, of course, the general and surgical hospital.

Since the term intermediate care and skilled nursing care are written into federal Medicare and Medicaid laws, your physicians will likely be familiar with them. Before shopping for a home, have your physician tell you whether your relative needs skilled or intermediate care. Remember that, as a rule of thumb, patients needing intensive medical or nursing care require skilled care, whereas those who need supervision and help with eating, dressing, and the like are likely to need intermediate care. Tell the administrator which level of care your loved one needs. A bed in the intermediate care section of a nursing home or a bed in a nursing home which offers nothing but intermediate care will cost less than a bed in a skilled nursing facility.

THE COST OF NURSING HOME CARE

Nursing home care is becoming increasingly expensive. At the present time, patients who pay their own way can expect an average of $800 a month. Those patients and families who want to pay their own way should shop around, compare prices, and make sure that the quoted price for care is all-inclusive. Many homes quote a basic rate which includes only bed and board, thereafter charging extra for every service they perform and every supply they provide from Kleenex to toothpaste. It is essential that families establish in detail what the monthly charges will be and that they secure in writing the administrator's agreement that the patients can continue receiving drugs from their own pharmacy.

But few seniors or their families can afford to pay for nursing home care. It is therefore important to re-emphasize what Medicare and Medicaid provide.

Medicare, which is available to all older Americans over 65, pays for only the most intensive level of nursing care, skilled nursing following a hospital stay. The rules for eligibility are presently so narrowly drawn that few people are eligible. If your loved one is in a hospital, physicians and hospital case workers can provide an educated guess as to whether your loved one would qualify for the Medicare nursing home benefit.

Medicaid is a federal-state program, and consequently eligibility varies from state to state. But generally, those with limited assets, perhaps $2,500 or less in cash or securities, are eligible. Medicaid will pay for both levels of care—skilled and intermediate—without reference to prior hospitalization. Assuming, for example, that the nursing home charges $500 a month and the patient has $200 in Social Security benefits or other income, these funds will be used to offset the nursing home charges. In most states, the patient will be allowed to retain $25 of his Social Security check as personal expense money. The remaining $175 would be applied to the $500 bill, with the state paying $325 a month. It is a violation of the law for the administrator or owner to charge the family (or patient) extra amounts over and above the sums paid by Medicaid.

Those who wish to learn more about the operation of the Medicare nursing home program should contact their local district Social Security office. To learn more about Medicaid, contact the local welfare office.

MAKING A SHOPPING LIST

As Thomas Routh of the Hillsborough Department of Public Welfare said, the senior citizen is carrying the cross when it comes to choosing a nursing home. Nursing homes are very much a blind item; they cannot be judged by appearances. Each home must be evaluated closely on its own merits. This involves two steps: first preparing a list and then making inspections.

Most state health or welfare departments publish a list of homes licensed by the state. This list gives you the added dividend of knowing a home is licensed, the name of the administrator, and generally the level of care offered by the home.

You may also obtain a list by calling your state nursing home association. Every state has affiliates of the American Association of Homes for the Aged and the American Health Care Association. The former represent nonprofit, church-sponsored facilities, and the latter represent for-profit homes. In Washington state, the affiliate of nonprofit homes, for example, is the Washington Association of Homes for the Aged. Normally, the for-profit organization would be called the Washington Nursing Home Association, but in this state, as in many others, for-profit organizations have purged the words nursing home. Accordingly, you would find the proprietary nursing home association under the Washington Health Facilities Association. Generally, these groups will have their offices in your state capitol.

If all else fails, make yourself a list from the yellow pages of the telephone book. If you do so, do not be impressed by the large ads or the representations they make about the home and its facilities. Take nothing for granted. You must verify everything for yourself.

Having a list in hand, the next step is to start weeding out those homes that are unacceptable. You will want to eliminate some homes that are too far away to permit visiting by friends or family. You must also consider the type of location. Only you will know whether your loved one prefers the city to the suburbs or the country. As much as possible, let the patient make the decision. Consult your local rabbi, priest, or minister for advice. They should be able to give you some tips about the home on your list and may suggest new ones.

You will also want your family physician's recommendation. You should also consult with your local hospital's social worker or case worker. It goes without saying that you should call your local chapter of the American Association of Retired Persons and the National Council of Senior Citizens. Similarly, many states and cities have watchdog or ombudsman organizations that you should contact, such as Citizens for Better Care in Detroit and the Minneapolis Age and Opportunity Center in the Twin Cities, Minnesota. Finally, you should visit your state department of health and ask to see the inspection files on several of the homes you are considering. Such information must be made available to the public under the terms of Section 249 C of Public Law 92-603.

What Time Should You Visit a Nursing Home?

Between seven and eight in the morning, when the shifts change and breakfast is being served, or between 11 a.m. and 1 p.m., when you can observe the noon meal, are the best times to observe home operation. A return visit late at night may often be very revealing. Some homes allow you to visit and inspect only during certain hours, and most often you will need an appointment to see the administrator. As a general rule, the more open the facility, the better the care. Be wary of homes that sharply limit visitations and refuse to let you see the entire home or refuse to let you see it a second time if you desire.

What to Look For in Your Shopping Visits

Armed with a little information and the right questions to ask, senior citizens and their families can make an intelligent choice of the nursing homes offering care in their area. Beginning with those homes that have survived your initial evaluation, you should begin your visits analyzing each component of the nursing home as if you were a trained detective. Again, take nothing for granted. Ask to see the nursing home's license. Make sure it is current. Beware of temporary or provisional renewals. And make sure the administrator has a license from the state indicating that s/he has the training for this important position. If Medicare or Medicaid is paying the bill, be certain that the home is eligible to participate in these programs.

Evidence of Human Dignity

First and foremost, look for the intangible, what Dr. Karl Menninger called "the spirit of the place." Observe how the patients are treated by the staff. All the staff from the janitor on up to the administrator should be genuinely interested in their patients. Do the patients look busy and happy? Are they treated with kindness and respect? Does the staff respond quickly to the patients' requests for help? Is there any evidence of efforts to preserve the patients' right of choice in all aspects of their daily living. Nothing is more destructive to morale than being regimented and told what to do at every turn. Is there evidence that the home is trying to help the patients maintain their identity? Are residents encouraged to bring their books, pictures, and other personal effects with them? Are patients free to come and go as they please? Does the home encourage visitors, and do they have liberal visiting hours?

Do patients have some degree of privacy? Are doors closed or screens installed when patients are given baths? Are men and women given a bath at the same time? What provisions does the home have for helping patients out of bathtubs or whirlpools? Are there machines for this or does the home rely on its maintenance man to help lift heavy women into or out of the bathtub?

Are patients dressed in clothes that are neat and clean, or are they wearing hospital gowns? Do the clothes seem to fit? Put differently, do the clothes appear to belong to the patients? Are they wearing stockings, shoes, or slippers? Are they well groomed? Are the men clean-shaven? Do the women have their hair done? Are their fingernails and toenails clean and trimmed?

Is there an isolation room for patients with infectious diseases or for the use of acutely ill or dying patients? Does the home have patients recently discharged from the state mental hospital? What sort of psychiatric care is provided for them? Are these or other disturbed patients placed in the same room with patients who are alert but physically ill?

Is there any evidence of racial or other types of segregation? Does the home provide the same food for private paying patients as they provide for welfare patients? Are welfare (Medicaid) patients or private patients placed in one wing of the facility?

The Physical Plant

Another important aspect in your investigation involves the physical plant and how it operates. But do not be misled into thinking that a new and modern nursing home will always provide the best care.

Many older buildings contain more than adequate systems. Once again, you must ask questions.

What does the outside of the home look like? Is it well kept and land-scaped? Is it constructed of brick, wood or other materials? When was it built? Was it built originally as a nursing home or converted? Are ad-ditions to the original structure evident? If so, do they have heat, elec-tricity and adequate fire protection? If the facility is more than one story, are there adequate fire escapes? What are they made of, and are they operable?

Evaluate the inside of the nursing home. Is plaster falling from the walls? Is there any water damage indicating the roof leaks? Has it been freshly painted? Has the home made effective use of color? Are there stains from urine or feces on the floor? If there is carpet on the floor, what is its flame spread rating and are there sprinklers in pa-tients' rooms as well as in the heating and laundry rooms? If the home has no sprinklers but it does have carpeting, then the carpet should be certified as having a flame spread score of 75 or less on the American Society of Testing and Materials E-84 Tunnel Test. Are the hallways wide enough to permit two wheel chairs to pass with ease and are there adequate handrails?

What are the conditions in the patient's rooms—especially the bathrooms? Is there a bathroom with a sink, toilet, and shower in every room? If not, how convenient are these facilities? If the facilities are shared, how many people use them? Are they clean and free from odors? Beware of aerosol perfumes, pine oil, or other masking odors. Good homes restore function to patients as soon as possible and attend to incontinent patients quickly, so odors do not permanently pollute the air. Are there grab bars around toilets and showers to aid pa-tients?

Are patients overcrowded? Are the beds comfortable? Is there a call system over every bed? Does it work? Are there call systems in bathrooms or showers? Are there reading lights for patients' beds? Are there lockers for the storage of belongings? Is there fresh water at bedside? Are there windows in patients' rooms?

What kind of heating and cooling system does the home have and how effective is it? Do the patients appear comfortable? Check the thermostat to see where it is set and take a temperature reading. Ideally, for the aged and infirm, it should read between 72 and 76 all year round. When was the home's last fire safety inspection? Ask to see their inspection report from the fire department. Check the elec-trical wiring. Are bare wires present? Are stairways enclosed and doors kept closed? When was the home's last fire drill? How often are they held? Are there written emergency plans in evidence? Are there ramps to accommodate wheel chair patients? Are exits clearly marked? Are these exit doors locked from the inside? Is the lighting in the home adequate? Check the wattage on the bulbs being used. Are burned out bulbs replaced? Does the facility cut back the heat or turn off the air conditioning at night?

Are common areas provided for socializing, lounging, or other activities? Are these rooms being used for the purpose specified? Is there equipment such as games, yarn, and paints to indicate that crafts are taking place? Is there a separate dining room? Is it attractive?

By all means, check more than one floor. The first floor and the lounge you see when you enter are sometimes given extra attention to attract new customers. The first floor is often called the show floor. You should check the second and third floors, where homes traditionally sequester their sickest patients.

Food Preparation

One of the most frequent complaints received by the Senate Committee on Aging is that the quality of food in nursing homes is generally inadequate in both quantity and quality. Happily, however, many nursing homes have excellent meal services. You will be able to tell at a glance which category your home falls into if you arrive at meal time. In analyzing food services, it is a good idea to start at the source — the kitchen.

Is the kitchen clean? Note the floors, the stoves, the refrigerator, the storage areas. Is there any evidence of insects or rodents? Does the home have an extermination service? How often do they visit? Evaluate the cleanliness of those preparing the food. Are they wearing hairnets and clean aprons? Do these people also perform maintenance work? Do they care for patients as well as work in the kitchen? In performing both functions, employees would run the risk of spreading infection. Have these kitchen employees had required tests for infectious diseases, including an x ray for tuberculosis? What provision is made for garbage disposal? Check the conditions in the alley behind the nursing homes where the garbage cans are traditionally stored.

Does the home have the services of a dietician? Who makes up the menu to ensure good nutrition? Does the food served on a particular day conform to what is posted on the menu? If not, why not? Are therapeutic diets being followed? Almost any home will have a few diabetics or others requiring special diets, e.g., salt free, low sodium or pureed. Are these special diets evident? Examine them, make sure that special diets are just that rather than the same meal received by the rest of the patients with a different color card marking it.

Is the food appetizing? Is it adequate in quantity? Is it recognizable? Does Spanish rice look like Spanish rice? Are warm things served warm and cold things served cold? Is it served in covered plates? Has the food been left sitting at room temperature during the process of preparation or prior to serving — particularly anything made with eggs or mayonnaise? How many meals are served each day and at what time? Do they allow plenty of time for the patients to eat? Do staff members feed those unable to feed themselves? Can patients have seconds? Are snacks served between meals and at bedtime?

The Home's Personnel and Their Nursing Services

The competency and attitude of the nursing staff obviously greatly affect the patients' well-being. Look for signs that there are enough trained employees to meet their needs, that these personnel have the necessary skills and the proper positive attitudes.

You might start with the administrator — after asking to see both the nursing home's license and the administrator's, ask about the administrator's experience. Is the administrator owner of this facility or a hired manager? What about other business interests? Is the administrator on the premises? How often and how long? Easily reached? Even on weekends? In emergencies?

Find out how many nurses the home employs full time and part time. Take down their names and check them against the nursing registry in your state. Both registered nurses and licensed practical nurses must be licensed by the state. An RN must have at least two years' special education. Make sure an RN is in charge in a skilled nursing facility seven days a week, eight hours a day. Preferably, the home you select will have an RN in charge of all three shifts — morning, afternoon, and evening. However, federal regulations require only a licensed practical nurse in charge of nursing on the afternoon and evening shifts. An LPN must have the minimum of one year's specialized training. ICFs require only one LPN in charge eight hours a day. Most of the employees in nursing homes are nurse's aides. They provide 80 to 90 percent of the care in nursing homes. These individuals should have completed four-week training courses for a minimum competency. Learn if the home provides such an in-service or other training program for aides as a precondition of their employment. Is there any effort to provide continuing education after they have been hired?

Check to see that only the licensed personnel, the RNs and LPNs, set up and pass medications. Avoid any homes where aides pass medication or have access to the medication and narcotics cabinet. Ascertain if the RNs spend much of their time caring for patients or if they are too busy with administrative duties such as ordering supplies, filling Medicare forms, and greeting visitors and prospective applicants.

Ask how much the nurse's aides are paid and how many of them there are. Do they know what to do in the case of an emergency? Do they have enough supplies to do their job, such as towels, toothpaste, a spa, bed pans, mops, and cleaners. What is the home's turnover rate? (How many aides did the home hire and lose in the past year as compared with the average number who serve the facility?) What is the home's ratio of personnel to patients? At the present time, U.S. nursing homes average 0.6 personnel for every one patient. Your home should have roughly the same number of employees overall as it has patients. If you are shown cards on a time clock as evidence of the number of employees, check to see how many of the cards are blank and how many are part time.

Ask the administrator how many full-time or part-time therapists are available to assist patients. Good homes provide speech therapy, occupational therapy, and physical therapy. Write down the names of these employees and check their credentials with the appropriate professional association.

Medical Services

Because the services of a competent medical staff are critical to the health and well-being of patients, you must learn if the nursing home has a medical director. What are the director's responsibilities? Is s/he simply the house doctor who treats patients without private physicians of their own, or does s/he assume responsibility for the medical care of the residents in the facility? As a rule, most nursing homes continue to expect patients' personal physicians to care for them in the facility. Try to learn who is responsible in emergencies. Learn what procedures are followed upon admitting a patient. Are patients given a physical examination and a medical order instituted immediately? How often do physicians visit the home? They should visit each patient at least once every 30 days. Learn also if the home has the services of a dentist or podiatrist and how often they visit the facility.

Find out how many incontinent and nonambulatory patients the home has. Most facilities are not anxious to accept these so-called heavy-care patients. The way these patients are treated often separates good homes from the bad. Do the patients have bedsores, indicating they have not been turned regularly? Are they left sitting in their own waste? Turn down a few made up beds and look for stains, or worse. Are many patients restrained? If so, how long are they tied up and with what are they tied? Are they restrained with torn sheets, leather straps, Posey belts, or by means of adult high chairs? Is there a physician's prescription to justify the use of the restraints?

Do the patients look sedated? Are they attentive or in a stupor? Are their feet swollen from constant sitting? Is there evidence they get exercise? If so, what kind? Can they walk on the grounds of the nursing home?

Check the medication cabinet. Narcotics should be kept in a locked container within the locked medications room. Are the drugs orderly so that it is easy to identify which drugs belong to patients? Look for evidence that the home retains left-over drugs belonging to dead or discharged patients. Beware of any home which keeps a box full of prescription containers with various names on them on the floor of the medications room. Is there any evidence that over-the-counter items have prescription labels on them, indicating the government might be paying for items the home is supposed to supply. Find out if the drugs are all supplied by the same pharmacy. Patients should have the right to retain their own pharmacies. Denial of this right often leads to inflated drug prices.

Find out if the nursing home has an agreement with a nearby hospital in case a patient becomes acutely ill. Ask the administrator if there is such a transfer agreement and with which hospital. If not, what course of action would the home follow in an emergency?

The Activities Program

Activities in nursing homes are essential to reducing patients' feelings of isolation. Without activities and recreation programs, a stay in a nursing home can be an unbearable experience. Proper activities integrated into the patients' overall regimen of care and therapy can be an invaluable asset to rehabilitating patients, improving their self-esteem and making their stay in a home pleasurable. Residents in St. Joseph's Manor in Trumbull, Connecticut have been heard to remark, "I am 82 years old and since my admission to this facility, I am just learning what it means to be alive and happy." In any activities program, it is important that patients be encouraged to participate, but they should not be forced to do so.

Analyze what activities are available, how they are utilized, and how well they are received by patients. Look for evidence that the activities listed are actually provided. Are there religious services? Have arrangements been made for the visits of priests, rabbis, and ministers? Are there social workers available to help patients and their families adjust to institutionalization, or to help with other personal problems? Do volunteers provide entertainment and instruction in arts and crafts? Is there anything for patients to do besides watch TV? Does the home have self-government, allowing the patients some voice in the operation of the facility and in the choice of activities? Are there birthday and anniversary remembrances and parties? Outside trips and excursions? In short, how many of the activities offered by the Iowa Soldiers' Home are offered by the home you are evaluating?

THE PATIENT'S BILL OF RIGHTS

As of October 3, 1974, the Department of Health, Education, and Welfare published regulations in the *Federal Register* which set forth a bill of rights for nursing home patients. It is important for you and your loved one to become familiar with each of these rights. In your visits to the facility before placement, try to see if these rights have been preserved for patients already in the facility. After placement of your relative in a facility, vigilantly check to make sure that these rights are not abridged in any way. The bill of rights which follows requires that each patient admitted to a facility:

1. Is fully informed, as evidenced by the patient's written acknowledgment, prior to or at the time of admission and during stay, of these rights and of all rules and regulations governing patient conduct and responsibilities;
2. Is fully informed, prior to or at the time of admission and during stay, of services available in the facility, and of related charges including any charges for services not covered under titles XVIII (Medicare) or XIX (Medicaid) of the Social Security Act, or not covered by the facility's basic per diem rate;
3. Is fully informed, by a physician, of his medical condition unless medically contraindicated (as documented by a physician, in his medical report), and is afforded the opportunity to participate in the planning of his medical treatment and to refuse to participate in experimental research;
4. Is transferred or discharged only for medical reasons, or for his welfare of that of other patients, or for non-payment for his stay (except as prohibited by titles XVIII or XIX of the Social Security Act), and is given reasonable advance notice to ensure orderly transfer or discharge, and such actions are documented in his medical record;
5. Is encouraged and assisted, throughout his period of stay, to exercise his rights as a patient and as a citizen, and to this end may voice

grievances and recommend changes in policies and services to facility staff and/or to outside representatives of his choice, free from restraint, interference, coercion, discrimination, or reprisal;

6. May manage his personal financial affairs, or is given at least a quarterly accounting of financial transactions made on his behalf should the facility accept his written delegation of this responsibility to the facility for any period of time in conformance with State law;

7. Is free from mental and physical abuse, and free from chemical and (except in emergencies) physical restraints except as authorized in writing by a physician for a specified and limited period of time, or when necessary to protect the patient from injury to himself or to others;

8. Is assured confidential treatment of his personal and medical records, and may approve or refuse their release to any individual outside the facility, except in case of his transfer to another health care institution, or as required by law or third-party payment contract;

9. Is treated with consideration, respect, and full recognition of his dignity and individuality, including privacy in treatment and in care for his personal needs;

10. Is not required to perform services for the facility that are not included for therapeutic purposes in his plan of care;

11. May associate and communicate privately with persons of his choice, and send and receive his personal mail unopened, unless medically contraindicated (as documented by his physician in his medical record);

12. May meet with, and participate in activities of social, religious, and community groups at his discretion, unless medically contraindicated (as documented by his physician in his medical record);

13. May retain and use his personal clothing and possessions as space permits, unless to do so would infringe upon rights of other patients, and unless medically contraindicated (as documented by his physician in his medical record); and

14. If married, is assured privacy for visits by his/her spouse; if both are in-patients in the facility, they are permitted to share a room, unless medically contraindicated (as documented by the attending physician in the medical record).[1]

What to Do If You Have a Complaint

Many elderly and their families are afraid to ask àll of the above questions for fear of alienating the nursing home administrator or staff. Those providers who are proud of their homes and with nothing to hide will welcome your full and thorough evaluation. Those who resist your efforts to examine their facilities closely should be ruled out. If you have a complaint about what you see in the course of shopping for a nursing home or about the care your loved one has received after entering a facility, you should first bring it to the attention of the administrator. If you fail to obtain satisfaction, then address a letter with all the specifics you can discover (names, dates, addresses, witnesses) to your senator or representative in Washington, D.C. Send a carbon copy of this letter to the director of your state department of health. (See Appendix C for a complete list of where to go for help.)

The members of the Senate and House Committees on Aging especially would welcome your letters and would do whatever they could to resolve the problems. If they cannot help, they will tell you so at once, and your recourse will be to engage a reputable lawyer or, if you have limited funds, to contact your local legal aid society.

While this chapter is written from the consumer's point of view, the advice to nursing home administrators is implied. The list of questions to aid consumers is little more than a restatement of current laws and requirements with respect to nursing homes. Facilities which are in compliance with federal and state standards have little to fear from a few probing questions. Indeed, the more open and honest administrators are with prospective clients, the more they will inspire confidence. If administrators want still more advice about what they can do to be attractive to seniors and their families, they might institute any or all of the several positive and innovative programs outlined in the preceding chapter.

Nursing home administrators should also be encouraged to write their elected representatives when they feel regulations are unfair, or to redress any other grievance. The House and Senate congressional committees will be receptive to hearing your point of view.

Part IV

Reforms

If virtue was profitable, common sense would make us good, and greed would make us saintly. And we'd live like the angels in the happy land that needs no heroes. But since, in fact, we see that avarice, anger, envy, pride, sloth, lust and stupidity commonly profit far beyond humility, chastity, fortitude, justice and thought, and have to choose, to be human at all... why then perhaps we MUST stand fast a little... even at the risk of being heroes.

> —*A Man For All Seasons*
> by Robert Bolt

Chapter 16

Suggestions for Improvement

Not surprisingly, there has been little agreement on the subject of nursing home reform. Some people suggest that bad nursing homes, like the poor, will always be with us. Others, who are equally negative, insist that nursing home problems have their roots in contemporary attitudes toward the aged in our society — attitudes which, they contend, are virtually impossible to change. Others offer slightly more hope, observing that nursing homes are today where hospitals were 30 years ago — meaning that with time come improvement and greater acceptance, even among institutions.

The simple fact is that societal attitudes can be changed and the quality of nursing home care can be improved. We need not wait 30 years; it can happen today. All that is needed is an aroused citizenry exerting continuous pressures on its elected representatives. Federal legislation is the quickest and most effective way of changing social attitudes.

We must attack the problem at many levels. We must find ways to work with honest nursing home administrators who want to band together to eliminate the bad apples from their midst. An effort must be made to educate operators and employees in the techniques of motivating patients. Society must hold in esteem those operators who run excellent programs.

Lack of a Policy Toward the Infirm Elderly

Chapter 9 is an in-detail discussion of the fact that the United States has not yet decided what it is going to do with its infirm elderly. No policy exists at the present time. There is, instead, only the hollow pretense of care and concern. Medicare's little blue handbook advertises that the government pays for nursing home care, but the fine print takes away what the big print gives. Reality does not follow rhetoric. Only 8,300 people out of the one million in nursing homes on any given day have their care paid for by Medicare.

The only federal assistance that is available is through Medicaid, the welfare nursing home program. Only the poor who are without income and who have exhausted their assets are eligible. Even so, Medicaid payments make up more than half of the industry's $10.5 billion revenues this year.

It is a sad commentary that despite these whopping expenditures, 600,000 older Americans each year are going without nursing home care. They simply cannot afford the services they need. By the same token, there are perhaps 2.5 million older Americans who are in need of home health services but who are doing without because of the lack of government commitment to these programs. Expenditures for home health care amounted to only about one percent of either Medicare or Medicaid last year.

All in all, the picture is one of great progress in the attention given to nursing homes by the community and in the efforts nursing homes are exhibiting to make life more worthwhile for their infirm residents. However, despite the new positive and innovative programs, there is still much room for improvement. These innovations must become the rule, rather than the isolated example. Good nursing homes must become better until the day that the negative image of nursing homes has been erased. On that day, children in America will be heard to say: "I want to be a nursing home administrator when I grow up."

The recommended reforms in this chapter are the natural correlatives of the root cause for nursing home problems detailed in Part II. For example, if the first major obstacle is the lack of a national policy toward the infirm elderly, then a policy must be established. If the present system offers financial incentives to poor care, those incentives must be reversed. If doctors and nurses have not always been sensitive to the needs of the ill elderly, then they must be sensitized. If existing laws and regulations are not being enforced because of political interference or for other reasons, then this too must change.

Congress must act quickly to fashion a national policy. A comprehensive package of benefits is needed which should be sufficiently flexible so as to permit the selection of an approach best suited to each person's needs. The following proposals should be considered.

—Broaden the scope of Medicare to provide comprehensive nursing home benefits to all needy Americans regardless of prior hospitalization or ability to pay. Nursing home benefits should be a matter of right for all, not a privilege grudgingly extended only to the elderly poor.

— Amend the Internal Revenue Code to allow a family to deduct as a medical expense payments made by a family for the nursing care of a relative (whether the relative qualifies as a dependent or not). This will allow more families to keep their elderly at home and enable them more easily to pay for the cost of a relative's nursing home stay.

— Authorize an experimental program to subsidize families to care for their elderly in their own homes. If we are willing to pay $800 a month to keep a patient in a nursing home under Medicaid, why not pay a family $150 a month to take care of that person at home?

— Broaden the scope of Medicare to provide greater availability of in-home services and to authorize the payment for adult day care. In more and more families, both husband and wife work; often they are afraid to leave an aged relative at home alone during the day. The result has too often been premature institutionalization. Day care would offer them the security of knowing a loved one was being cared for by day and allow them to have the pleasure of the relative's company through the dinner and evening hours.

— Modify the Medicare reimbursement formula so that small hospitals in rural areas with chronic low vacancy rates can provide nursing home care where there are no appropriate nursing home beds available. Too many small towns are issuing bonds to build municipal nursing homes while their local hospitals are in financial trouble with more than half of their beds idle.

— Allow the use of Supplementary Security Income payments plus a state supplement to house residents in shelter care facilities which meet certain federal minimum standards. This proposal is designed to encourage the states to regulate the unlicensed boarding homes referred to in Chapter 6.

Financial Incentives to Poor Care

Some 80 percent of America's 23,000 nursing homes operate for profit. However, the structure of Medicare and Medicaid reimbursement formulas encourages them to cheat. Under a flat rate, $20 or $25 a day, operators know that the only way to make a profit is to cut back on food or nursing. In a cost-plus system, they know the object is to run up reimbursable costs, so large salaries are paid, relatives are put on the payroll, and inflated rents are paid to related corporations. This system also encourages trading in real estate — selling nursing homes back and forth, since operators are reimbursed on equity, which in turn is determined by the selling price of a home.

In both systems there is a fundamental contradiction between the patient's prime interest (returning home) and that of the operator, who needs to keep beds filled. Under both systems, bed-bound patients bring a higher rate of reimbursement than ambulatory patients. There is no incentive to rehabilitate patients.

Congress must tie Medicare and Medicaid reimbursement formulas to the quality of care provided. The financial incentives must be lined up in the direction of good care. One suggestion calls for judging nursing homes on two levels: capability and actual performance. Under such a system, nursing homes would be graded on their ability to meet or exceed standards. They would also be graded on the care that they provide. A medical review team composed of physicians, nurses, dieticians, and social workers would review the performance of the home against reasonable expectations and its progress in meeting therapeutic goals outlined at the time of each patient's admission.

Sensitizing Physicians

Physicians have failed to pay attention to the needs of nursing home patients. As a result, the quality of medical care in nursing homes is less than adequate. One of the primary reasons for physician disinterest in nursing homes is the lack of emphasis on aging and long term care in American medical schools.

Congress should deal with this problem by making federal funds available to establish departments of geriatrics in schools of medicine. Geriatrics is given special emphasis in England and Scandinavia, but not in the United States. This oversight should be corrected so that future generations of physicians will take notice of the unique medical and social problems confronting the ill aged.

Congress should also make funds available to train discharged medics and physician assistants in geriatrics and the needs of nursing home patients. If physicians are unable to carry the full load of caring for the elderly in nursing homes, paramedical personnel working under their direction can provide day-to-day supervision.

Training for Nurses and Other Personnel

Schools of nursing are just beginning to devote their attention to the special problems of the infirm aged. There is a strong desire to expand training in geriatrics and gerontology. Accordingly, Congress should make funds available:

- to establish graduate programs for nurses in geriatrics and gerontology. Many nurses would like to specialize in this way but have no opportunity to do so at the present time.
- to place increased emphasis on the training of nurse practitioners in geriatrics so that they may provide primary care in nursing homes. Registered nurses with additional training can perform many of the routine, chronic maintenance procedures needed by patients in long term care facilities.
- to institute continuing education programs for nurses in geriatrics. Many nurses who graduated some time ago would like to return to schools for an update on the latest developments in the care of the aged.
- to provide expanded in-service training programs for nursing home personnel. There is little federal support for such programs at present. This is unfortunate in view of the fact that aides and orderlies provide 80 to 90 percent of the care in nursing homes.

Proposals to Help Nursing Homes Upgrade

Many nursing homes cannot obtain financing needed to secure improvements or renovations. In other cases, church groups and non-profit agencies have been unable to obtain financing to build nursing homes in areas of great need. Three proposals are suggested including bills:

- authorizing direct loans for the construction and rehabilitation of nursing homes owned and operated by churches or other non-profit agencies. Loans would be obtained from the government at a moderate interest (perhaps 4 percent) and repayable over a long term (perhaps 50 years).
- authorizing grants for the planning, development, construction and rehabilitation of nursing homes in black or minority communities. Such extraordinary assistance is needed to bring facilities into areas where the most needy live.
- authorizing the liberalization of FHA Section 232 which provides FHA insurance to aid in the construction of nursing homes. Homes with excellent performance records should also be able to secure insured loans for renovations.

New Standards for Nursing Homes

HEW has never fully implemented the Moss amendments of 1967. Consequently, many federal standards contemplated by Congress have never been issued. Compounding the problem, HEW in 1974 issued unified standards for nursing homes participating in both Medicare and Medicaid. However, HEW ignored a congressional directive stating that if the rules of the two programs were in conflict, the highest standard should be retained in every case. Inexplicably, HEW weakened the standards in many respects. Some of the losses were prevented because of Senate hearings, but others were not. Congress must now act to restore needed standards and provide necessary protections to patients.

— Require physician visits at least once every 30 days. Present rules allow 60-day intervals — or longer in the case of intermediate care facilities — between visits.

— Require skilled nursing homes participating in Medicare and Medicaid to have at least one RN on duty 24 hours a day, seven days a week. Studies indicate the quality of care increases directly with the number and proportion of RNs on the nursing staff. Some state laws are much tougher, requiring one RN for every 30 patients.

— Require that only RNs be permitted to set up and pass medications in skilled nursing homes. As indicated, there is a significant problem with the poor administration of drugs in nursing homes. Average drugs administered in error drop dramatically with the number of RNs on duty.

— Require HEW to promulgate minimum ratios between nursing personnel and patients. Each patient should receive no less than 2.25 hours of nursing time per day. This was an existing federal standard deleted in 1974. Under present federal rules, all that is required in nursing homes, *no matter what their size,* is one RN seven days a week on the morning shift and one LPN on each of the afternoon and evening shifts.

— Require that nursing homes provide medically related social services. This is another provision that was deleted by a short-sighted administration.

— Require admission contracts between the nursing home and the patient, and prohibit life-care contracts. Unhappily, there are still reports of patients' being required to sign over their homes or their life savings in return for nursing home care, supposedly to the end of their days. If a patient lives long, the home may feel cheated; if the patient dies quickly, relatives or the estate may feel swindled.

—Require nursing home administrators promptly to report and treat epidemic diseases, accidents, and significant changes in patient conditions. Too often, operators have failed to report outbreaks of flu or salmonella until it was too late. Families also complain that they are not informed until several days after a loved one has an accident.

—Require nursing homes to file CPA-audited cost and financial statements. And provide penalties for fraud or misrepresentation. Operators, in effect, would have to certify the truthfulness of their request for reimbursement from federal programs.

—Require full and complete disclosure of nursing home ownership. Present laws are full of loopholes so that it is virtually impossible to tell who owns nursing homes in any state.

The Enforcement Effort

As indicated in previous chapters, there are numerous shortcomings related to the enforcement of nursing home regulations. Following are a dozen recommended changes in the law to facilitate a more realistic enforcement effort.

—Require unannounced inspections of nursing homes at least once every 90 days. Several states already insist on inspections more frequently than once a year. Also, require that state inspectors who conduct federal Medicare and Medicaid inspections have minimum qualifications and training. Some states were using state police for the job, and one was employing retired military personnel with no background in health for this purpose. Standardized training and qualifications are needed.

—Require HEW to establish a rating system for nursing homes as a guide to consumers.

—Provide strict new controls on the handling of patients' funds. Such funds are greatly misused at present. Most often, they are mingled with the home's operating revenues.

—Outlaw the practice of requiring patients to make a gift or other payment to the facility as a precondition of admitting them as Medicare or Medicaid patients.

—Provide warning on Medicaid forms that fraud or misstatements of a material fact in conjunction with the program is a federal crime. Defendants in federal cases have claimed they did not intend to violate federal law. They argue that they thought Medicaid was strictly a state program. Since at least half of the funds are federal, they should be deprived of this argument.

— Call upon HEW to establish a central clearinghouse of information on nursing home investigations. Many states have underway investigations which cross state lines. HEW is the natural agency to coordinate these efforts and to develop a central index of nursing home ownership.

— Clarify conditions under which federal funds can be withheld and Medicaid/Medicare certification revoked from individual nursing homes. Present authority is confused. Neither operators nor program administrators are sure of what happens.

— Provide 100 percent funding to the states to underwrite the cost of Medicare/Medicaid nursing home audits. There are few audits at the present time. States use lack of funds as an excuse. One benefit to the government will be that at least half of the money identified as overpayments by the auditors will be returned to the federal government.

— Make it a misdemeanor for anyone to exert pressure or otherwise cause a nursing home inspector to alter reports or otherwise provide preferential treatment to any nursing home. This may help slow down political interference.

— Create a cadre of federal inspectors to conduct spot checks of Medicare and Medicaid facilities to test the quality of state inspections. Experience has proven we can no longer rely totally upon state inspections.

— Authorize Medicare/Medicaid patients (or their guardians) to bring class actions against nursing homes which do not meet standards, offer poor care, or endanger the lives of residents. Giving patients direct access to injunctions in federal court may be the most effective deterrent to poor care and abuse in the long run.

TOWARD A NATIONAL POLICY: PROGNOSIS GOOD

Each of the foregoing proposals were introduced by Senator Moss early in 1975 as part of a 48-bill reform package. Representative Claude Pepper, chairman of the House Committee on Aging, introduced the same series of bills in the House of Representatives. Various bills have been reintroduced in 1977 by Mr. Pepper and Senators Frank Church and Edward M. Kennedy.

The bills were not offered casually. They were the result of some 25 hearings over six years and more than 3,000 pages of testimony compiled by the Subcommittee on Long Term Care. After the bills were introduced, the subcommittee held more than 14 hearings on nursing homes and related Medicaid abuses. Ten reports were issued, most of them dealing directly with nursing homes.

Of the original 48-bill package, only four were enacted by the time Congress adjourned in October 1976. Two amendments involving small amounts of federal funds were added to the Nurse Training Act, which passed the Senate on April 10, 1975. They authorize federal funds to schools of nursing to institute in-service training programs for nursing home personnel and to begin training nurse practitioners in geriatrics and the needs of nursing home patients. A third enacted proposal updated federal fire safety requirements for nursing homes.

The last bill created the Office of Inspector General in the Department of Health, Education and Welfare. This was a primary recommendation after the subcommittee's investigation of fraud and abuse in Medicaid mills. During this investigation, Senator Moss posed as a Medicaid patient and personally experienced the feeling of being "run through the mill."

Why didn't the other bills pass and what is the prognosis for the future? There are several reasons, including opposition by the administration, pressure from industry, and lack of interest on the part of legislative committees.

Neither the Senate nor the House aging committees has legislative authority. Their findings and the bills they originate must be referred to other committees. Most bills relating to nursing homes are referred to the Finance Committee in the Senate and to the Ways and Means Committee in the House. Neither of these has shown much interest in the topic until 1977. (Senator Herman Talmadge and Congressmen Dan Rostenkowski and Paul Rogers have introduced major fraud and abuse legislation which affects nursing homes.) In fairness, it should be pointed out that they have their hands full dealing with income tax reform, trade legislation, social security, and other matters. Moreover, strong pressure was exerted on the committees by the states and industry representatives against some of the proposals. However, the balance of the bills were publicly supported by the American Health Care Association, which represents for-profit nursing homes.

The more important opposition in this case came from the Ford administration, which opposed virtually all of the 48 bills. It opposed legislation making expanded nursing homes, day care, and expanded home health benefits available on the basis of its cost to the Treasury. It supported the concept of providing financial incentives to good care but claimed it will take years to implement the concept. It opposed training physicians, nurses, and aides in geriatrics and the needs of nursing home patients, claiming existing programs adequately meet the need. It refused to reinstate deleted standards and opposed more agressive enforcement efforts, claiming nursing homes were over-regulated.

President Ford made much of the overregulation of nursing homes in the course of his efforts to win the Texas presidential primary. On April 29, 1976, he told a cheering group of owners and operators belonging to the Texas Nursing Home Association:

> I likewise know that your organization has raised a good many questions about HEW's 1972 regulations.... It does appear to me — and I have talked to the Secretary of HEW about it — that there is an overzealous interference attempted by those regulations, and I hope we can do something affirmatively to change them.

The president's suggestion to retreat even from existing anemic standards summarizes his administration's attitude toward nursing home reform. His remarks should be viewed in the context of his refusal to accept the advice of his own advisory council and the dismal record of the Nixon-Ford administration with respect to problems affecting the elderly in general.

On March 31, 1975, the Federal Council on Aging issued their report to the president, urging him to take action on a number of critical issues. One chapter of the report is related to nursing homes and reads, in part, "The Council urges legislative action to develop high standards of safety and care in nursing homes. At the same time, it is essential that assistance be provided to enable facilities to meet such standards, especially those homes serving minorities and the poor." In his communication of July 27, 1975, the president responded, "The enforcement of these standards [nursing homes] is one of my Administration's highest priorities."

Addressing the Senate one day later, Senator Moss challenged this notion, saying that nursing home standards were "one of this Administration's lowest priorities. The president's statement reads as if he believes HEW has a sterling record in enforcing nursing home standards and that nothing further need to be done. Only incredible myopia and insensitivity to the most devastating of human needs would support that point of view." Senator Moss ended his remarks by asking for a presidential initiative on nursing homes, "to make up for the last 8 years of inaction by HEW."

Senator Church stated that the Ford administration was "rapidly establishing one of the most negative records on aging of any that I can remember." On September 28, 1976, Senator Edward M. Kennedy sounded the same theme: "Neglect for the Nation's elderly, disinterest in their needs, and a total absence of caring; that has been the record of the Ford Administration."

There is little doubt that we are at the cross-roads with respect to nursing homes. If reform comes, it must come in the Ninety-fifth Congress. If no action is taken, we will have lost the best opportunity that we ever had to remove this blight from the American conscience.

With a new administration in the White House, the outlook is good. President Jimmy Carter has expressed commitment to solving the problems confronting the elderly. He has expressed his interest to reform the Medicaid program, which provides the lion's share of nursing home expenditures.

In the final analysis, the choice is up to us. If we continue our bankrupt policy toward the aged, there is little doubt that nursing home problems will return in amplified form to haunt us and future generations. We must decide the parameters of our commitment to our elders. They deserve to know what they can expect from us. We must join together in political action to bring about legislative and administrative reform and to awaken the conscience of the nation.

Our alternative is to continue carrying the monstrous burdens of our guilt and fears.

Appendix A
The History of Old Age

In the past, few people lived long, at least by current standards. While there was great variation from society to society, those who did survive generally could count on sufficient food and a roof over their heads. Through force of custom, political power, property rights, or family rights, the elderly received their measure of respect until they became very old and ill. The aged and decrepit could expect one of four policies: (a) veneration to the end of their days, (b) some choice in their disposition, (c) abandonment or quarantine from society in general, or (d) gerocide (the killing of the aged). Whatever the policy, it was expected. The U.S. has no consistent policy toward the infirm elderly. The rhetoric speaks of care and concern, but the reality most closely compares with the abandonment practiced by so many primitive societies.

TREATMENT OF THE AGED AND INFIRM IN PRIMITIVE SOCIETY

Our knowledge of primitive societies and the way they treated their elderly is extremely limited, making any generalization dangerous. Nevertheless, a few universally accepted facts are inescapable. To begin with, few people lived to an advanced age, at least in our terms. Leo Simmons in his classic work "The Role of the Aged in Primitive Society" examined the attitudes of 71 primitive societies from the Aztecs of Mexico to the Xosa in Africa, concluding that the proportion of individuals age 65 and over in primitive societies rarely exceeds three percent. Where life is savage and brutal, survival is for the swift and strong.

Within the harshness of their basic circumstances, however, it is interesting to note the wide latitude in the treatment primitive societies accorded their elderly. Examples abound in the work of Simmons and the studies of Dr. Paul Hoch and Dr. Joseph Zubin, who wrote that the Australian aborigines of the River Darling watched over their old and infirm. The young people of the tribe followed them in their wanderings to make sure no harm would come to them. The Dieri of Australia also accorded respect to their elderly, as did the Ainu of Japan. Similarly, the Basonga of West Africa cared for their seniors even in very advanced old age. The Bongo of the Southern Sudan treated the mentally ill with respect but were less charitable towards the aged.

Indian tribes of the American northeast—the Iroquois, the Mohicans, Hurons, and others—respected old people and treated them well. The Pima of Southern California, on the other hand, reportedly threw stones at them to see them behave like children.[1]

The Hopi, for all their emphasis on physical fitness, placed a high premium on old age. Aged Eskimos were well treated, as were the Kwakiutl old people. From what we can tell, the Incas went to great lengths to provide for the sick and the aged. In Inca society, all citizens were bound to till the soil. The land designated to the gods was tilled first, then the land of the aged and infirm. Citizens cultivated their own plots last.

Which prerogatives sustained individuals furthest along in life? According to Leo Simmons,[2] first and foremost is kinship, family membership. Most societies shared food, but relatives ate first—particularly among hunters, fishers, and collectors, societies in which food was scarce. In more developed agricultural and herding societies with property rights, trade, and grain storage, supplying food to the hungry aged took on more of the aspect of an organized charity. The elderly often had the benefit of taboos, which ensured that they would be given certain portions of the animal to eat; it was believed that eating these items would be harmful to all but the aged. Among the Crow, entrail and bone marrow were reserved for the elderly. The Pomo of the Southwest reserved the eating of worms and caterpillars for the aged. The elderly Polar Eskimo was given exclusive rights to eat eggs, the heart, liver, and lungs. Internal organs are the most common subjects of food taboos. The Aztecs had an interesting taboo. They severely punished drunkeness, but those over 70 were exempt. Drinking was a privilege of age.

Property rights were great insurance that the aged would be fed and taken care of in primitive societies. This is true primarily because such property rights did not depend on physical prowess, but on the community's customs or laws, which were enforced with appropriate sanctions. In primitive societies, as in the present day, there was a big gap between those who grew old with property and those who grew old without it. Simmons observes, "To 'get capital' would have to be the most apt slogan for old age security almost anytime anywhere and for everyone."

Simmons also suggests that security for the aged depended on their wits. Many elders found politics and judicial affairs fruitful fields of endeavor. By exercising the role of judge, lawmaker, or medicine man, those who had property found they could preserve their hold on it. These roles became more available as societies developed more advanced economies and integrated social patterns.

The elderly especially laid claim to the medicine man role, becoming repositories of knowledge and magic—mediators with the supernatural. This put them in the catbird seat with supervisory rights at all the great events of life: childbirth, child naming, initiations, weddings, and funerals. This function made them directors of life's emergencies, keepers of tradition, and chief conservators of the status quo. Some writers have suggested this hold continued after death because of the widespread belief in ancestor worship.

If a generalization is permissible, it seems that in most societies the aged were reasonably well cared for and received their share of respect—at least until they were very ill and decrepit. Such individuals faced the threat of indifference or neglect. Of the 39 societies for which some data were available, Simmons notes that 18 practiced abandonment. The Crow, for example, left their very old and ill to die. The Xosa left them in the bush. The Creek gave them the choice between abandonment and voluntary death. The Omaha abandoned their elderly on the prairie. However, the fear of ghosts and possible disfavor with their gods motivated them to provide the discarded elderly with a camp site and some provisions.

The fear of ghosts and retribution caused similar mollification of the policy of abandonment practiced by so many other primitive societies. Bushmen in Africa built separate shelters for the aged and infirm. The Hottentots had separate huts set aside for the ill aged to whom they gave a piece of meat and an ostrich shell full of water. This approach was taken even by the Ainu of Japan, who venerated the elderly until the end of life. The very old were placed in isolated huts and fed until they died. Thereafter, the huts were burned and sent to heaven after them; more specifically, this was so that the spirits of old women would not return to haunt the village.

In some societies, such as the Eskimo, the elderly themselves had the responsibility, when they were no longer useful and food was in short supply, to walk out into the snow and perish. In other societies they were killed. This killing was viewed differently by different societies. In some, the killing of the aged was an honor, anticipated or even requested by the aged themselves. In others, it was regarded as outright murder. Still other societies practiced passive euthanasia— food and medicines were withdrawn. Some few societies took care of their old until they died. The nomadic Chippewa carried them on their backs wherever they wandered. Similar care was required among the Tallensi of Africa's Ivory Coast; to fail to do so was to become a nonperson, to incur the censure of society and the wrath of the ancestors.[3]

If another generalization can be made, it is that despite the diversity in treatment of the aged and ill in primitive societies, the particular procedure employed by the society was understood by all. The elderly knew the rules of the game. This kind of honesty and predictability in the treatment of the infirm elderly is absent in contemporary American society.

THE TREATMENT OF THE AGED
AND INFIRM IN EARLY CIVILIZATIONS

The Ancient Hebrews

Many writers have speculated about how the ancient Hebrews treated their elders. Most begin with the observation that the treatment of the elderly varied a great deal between the 14th and the 10th centuries B.C. The image of the desert patriarch who provided for an extended household of wives, children, and other relatives, servants and strangers comes immediately to mind. In this situation, respect for the aged, especially the patriarch, was essential; it helped guarantee survival in a desolate environment.[4]

Many authors note that in reality the passage of time did little to erode the respect accorded Hebrew elders. Proponents of this theory point to the Bible and the command, "Despise not thy mother when she is old and Honor thy Father and Mother that thine own days be long," as evidence for their case. It is no coincidence, they argue, that Jehovah was conceptualized as a kind, but stern, old man whose every word was law.

Koller, for example, writes that old age was inseparably linked with respect, power, and mysticism among the ancient Hebrews. Long life was viewed as a blessing rather than a burden. Once again turning to the Bible, he points out that those who received God's special attention and favor were given the gift of longevity: Methuselah was given 969 years, Noah 950 years, and Seth 912 years.

He adds that aging was equated with wisdom, and its symbol was the grey beard. Old men, in fact, were called "Zaken," a derivative of "Zakan," meaning "beard." Even when senility set in, the elders were still respected according to rabbinic teaching. Koller notes that the Talmudic scholars emphasize that not only the two perfect tablets of the Laws were placed in the ark, but also the broken fragments of the original Law, destroyed by Moses when he observed that his people were worshipping the golden calf. "In symbolism, the ever-probing Talmudic scholars found a parallel to respect for the aged, even if only the fragments of a once-great talent remained." "Death was explained as the 'divine punishment' for disobedience against a heaven sent directive in the Garden of Eden." It was not until the New Testament that "the original Hebraic disposition on death was transmuted to mean a possible chance for eternal life in an ethereal heaven."

Old Age in Ancient Greece

It is generally acknowledged that old age was venerated among the Greeks, although there was great variation from century to century and within the confines of each individual city state. Moreover, the preoccupation of the Greeks with youth and beauty has led some writers to conclude that there was a great gap between the ideal of treatment of the elderly and the actual practice. Koller, for example, looks at the way old age is portrayed in the literature and concludes that respect for the aged was honored more in the breach.

In point of fact, the Greeks recognized the loss of mental agility in old age and despised the physical limitations that old age represented. In some ways, the attitude of the Greeks is aptly summarized in Ben Franklin's statement, "All would live long but none would be old." Old age was desired by all, but when it came, it was viewed with animosity because it brought maladies. The inevitability of old age was accepted as part of the normal scheme of things, but it was hoped old age would pay as brief a visit as possible. The ideal was to decline so gradually as to be hardly perceptible; memory, intellect, and health should fade in the sunset, thought the Greeks, not drop off a sharp chasm.

While the Greeks did not necessarily look forward to old age, it is the concensus of the literature that the elders were treated with kindness and respect. From the earliest Homeric stories, the Greek word for elder, "Geron," was a title of respect. In addition, the Greek word, "*Presbevian*," to be older, also means to honor (i.e., to treat as an elder) and to be an ambassador.[5]

According to the literature, the best thing Greeks could do to gain the favor of the gods was to take care of their mothers and fathers in their old age. To fail to do so would bring dishonor to the family and injure the reputation of the ancestors. It has been stated by several writers that valiant performances in war were a means of honoring one's parents. In *Old Age Among the Ancient Greeks*, Bessie Richardson writes that among the Greeks, it was an offense punishable by a year in prison to strike a parent, to refuse to maintain an indigent parent or to neglect the duty of burial.

Under the laws of Solon, a legitimate son who failed to care for his parents in old age was tried and if convicted, lost his citizenship. Recognizing these facts, Richardson comments:

> In their attitude toward the aged and orphans we see the most redeeming feature of the Greeks. To find legislation in regard to the maintenance and treatment of parents is unusual. In less civilized races this deference to age might be construed as due to fear—to the uncanny sentiment connected with old age. But in people of so high a degree of culture it might be the result rather of mildness and good manners.

She adds that while not looking forward to death, the Greeks did recognize that old age offered certain advantages. Among these were calmness, an inner peace, and judgment—"the intellectual qualities of prudence, discretion and mature judgment were the natural heritage of old age and it was the duty of the old to impart to the young." It was for this reason that those over 50 were called upon to address the assembly first. In Sparta, the legislative body was the "Gerousia," the elders, who played a large role in government. Richardson summarizes:

> All great and good men have been affectionate towards their aged parents, realizing that they soon might be called upon to share their infirmities. All nations that have lived long or whose culture has experienced a potent influence have shared this spirit. Not only have the Greeks not been an exception to this rule, but they seem to have a peculiar pre-eminence in this respect.

Old Age Among the Romans and the Influence of the Church

Far too many writers have tied the Roman view of old age to the writings of Terrence, who wrote that old age is a disease. Likewise,

Seneca is repeatedly quoted as saying that old age is an incurable disease. The imitation of Greek traditions, according to some writers, extended not only to language, religion, and philosophy, but also to their wavering position between an official policy of good will toward the aged and the more practical unconcern for those individuals past their prime. Koller, for example, writes that the citizen soldier between 19 and 47 dominated Roman life and that older and younger citizens were comparatively disadvantaged.

Other writers accuse their contemporaries of confusing the way the Romans themselves viewed old age and the way that they treated their elders. Robert de Ropp suggests that the Romans more than the Greeks expected wise counsel from their elders. In fact, the word "Senate" or "Senatus" means "an assembly of senes or elders."[6] In Rome, it was this collection of elders, the Senate, that guided the ship of state. Young men for action, old men for counsel, is an admonition of Cicero, who also wrote, "It is not by miracles, speed or physical dexterity that great things are achieved, but by reflection; in those qualities, old age is usually not poorer but even richer."[7]

There is little doubt that the Roman law invested the aged with considerable power and authority. The pater familias, patria potestas and manus—the head of the family, the power of the father, and the hand of the husband over the wife were examples of such investiture.

Koller notes that in later Roman times, Christian writers such as St. Augustine were greatly preoccupied with the next life and thus gave little attention to the plight of the aged on earth. However, their influence led to the establishment of hospitals in which the poor, blind, sick, and the aged could be given medical treatment.

As the years went by, the development of the Cannon Law proved to be a great boon to the aged. The church's sincere dedication to saving souls was not limited to the rich, the well, or the young. Moreover, the church taught that wealth and power were merely transitory and should be shared if the owners hoped for salvation. Thus, charity and hospitality became part of medieval parish life, and many elderly found comfort in time of need. For those without friend or family, there was a new institution—the monastery—which provided food, clothing and shelter. As Koller notes, what appears to be most significant is that "the identification of poverty with infamy was unheard of before the 16th century; indeed the poorer a man was, the more Christlike he seemed."[8]

AGING IN AMERICA:
EVOLUTION OF THE NURSING HOME

Aging in Early America

Survival in colonial America demanded strong, healthy adults; it tended to exclude the very young and the very old. To make matters tougher for the aged, the first settlers brought with them from their native England the strict Calvinist doctrine embodied in Puritan traditions. Poverty and illness were viewed as punishment from a vengeful God.[9] Accordingly, the philanthropic principle of charity toward the aged and indigent was slow to develop in America.

In 1751, the first hospital, the Pennsylvania Hospital, was founded. It was followed soon thereafter by Philadelphia General, New York Hospital, and Bellvue Hospital. Each of these facilities had a poor house or almshouse as its progenitor. About this time, statutes were enacted to the effect that each city was responsible for the care of the poor and indigents within its borders. This increased the number of poor houses and resulted in the common practice of citizens' forcing the poor out of town. Accordingly, those without assets or family most generally joined transient bands drifting from town to town.

The choice between lodging in an almshouse and nomadic scrounging was a desperate one.[10] It wasn't until the latter part of the 19th century that any thought was given to reforming institutions for the sick and aged. In 1873, Connecticut established a state board of charities, but there was no clear line of demarcation identifying the purposes of almshouses, workhouses, poor houses, asylums, and hospitals until World War I. Early in the 20th century all of these terms were in use. They were the only home for thousands of aged and infirm.

Because of the bad conditions in these so-called "poor houses," which were generally public facilities, social pressures in the 1920s began to force them out of existence. The suggested reform was to move individuals from the public, and generally wretched facilities, into private homes — what might today be called foster care homes.

While many advocates during this time had suggested the need for a facility between the home and the hospital, the great impetus for the concept of proprietary nursing homes came as part of the Social Security Act of 1935. In reaction to the conditions of the public poor houses, Congress mandated that old age assistance funds under the act would not be made available to individuals housed in public institutions. The result was a tremendous growth in the numbers of private, for-profit boarding homes wherein individuals could receive old age assistance.

In the intervening years more facilities began offering some form of nursing and medical care in addition to board and room. But it was not until World War II that the licensing of nursing homes and convalescent care facilities became the common practice.

By the mid 1950s, the number of nursing facilities had grown significantly. The major reason was the increased life expectancy of senior citizens and their greater numbers. Changing social patterns and attitudes also were evident by the passage of the Kerr-Mills law in 1960. Undoubtedly, the greatest boost of all came in 1965 when Congress enacted the Medicare and Medicaid programs, changing nursing homes from an enterprise to an industry.

This book describes the system as it operates today. The shape of long term care facilities and the role they will play in the future depends on the American public. In the final analysis, nursing homes will become what we demand they become.

NOTES

1. Grune and Stratton, *Psychopathology of Aging* (New York: 1961).

2. The following paragraphs are paraphrased from Leo W. Simmons, *The Role of the Aged in Primitive Society* (New Haven: Yale University Press, 1945).

3. Meyer Fortes, *The Web of Kinship Among the Tallensi* (London: Oxford University Press, 1949).

4. The best book in this area is Marvin R. Koller, *Social Gerontology* (New York: Random House), upon which this section extensively relies.

5. See Bessie Richardson, *Old Age Among the Ancient Greeks* (Baltimore: Johns Hopkins University Press, 1933).

6. Robert S. de Ropp, *Man Against Aging* (New York: St. Martin's Press, 1960).

7. Cicero's classic work on aging is "De Senectute."

8. Koller, *op. cit.*

9. *Ibid.*

10. *Ibid.*

REFERENCES

Observations and quotations in this section liberally borrowed from the following texts:

Baird, Janel H., ed. *These Harvest Years*. New York: Doubleday, 1951.

de Ropp, Robert S. *Man Against Aging*. New York: St. Martin's Press, 1960.

Fortes, Meyer, *The Web of Kinship Among the Tallensi*. London: Oxford University Press, 1949.

Howell, Trevor H. *Our Advancing Years*. Phoenix, London, 1953.

Hill, Margaret Neville. *An Approach to Old Age and Its Problems*. Edinburgh and London: Oliver and Boyd, 1961.

Kellam, Constance. *A Literary Bibliography on Aging*. New York: Council on Social Work, Education, 1968.

Koller, Marvin R. *Social Gerontology*. New York: Random House, 1968.

Luth, Paul. *Geschichte der Geriatrie*. Stuttgart: Ferdinand Enke Verlag, 1965.

Richardson, Bessie. *Old Age Among the Ancient Greeks*. Baltimore: Johns Hopkins University Press, 1933.

Roberts, Nesta. *Our Future Selves*. London: Allen and Unwin, 1970.

Shock, Nathan. *A Classified Bibliography of Gerontology and Geriatrics*. Stanford: Stanford University Press, 1951.

Selected References on Aging: An Annotated Bibliography. Washington, D.C.: GPO, 1951.

Simmons, Leo W. *The Role of the Aged in Primitive Society*. New Haven: Yale University Press, 1945.

Tibbitts, Clark, ed. *Handbook of Social Gerontology, Societal Aspects of Aging*. Chicago: University of Chicago Press, 1960.

Townsend, Peter. *The Last Refuge*. London: Routledge and Kegan Paul, 1962.

Walker, Kenneth. *Commentary on Age*. London: Jonathan Cape, 1952.

Wolff, Kurt. *The Biological, Sociological, and Psychological Aspects of Aging*. Springfield, Ill.: Charles C. Thomas, 1959.

Zubin, Joseph and Hoch, Paul, eds. *Psychopathology of Aging.* New York: Grune and Stratton, 1961.

Appendix B
Advice to Nursing Home Administrators

With the hope that owners and administrators, as well as the general public, might gain full value from this book, we have included the following section of helpful hints, keyed to individual chapters of this book.

Chapter 1
Nursing Homes: The Greatest Fear of the Elderly

It goes without saying that nursing homes should do everything that they can to quiet the fears of the elderly. To begin with, providers can do much to allay the fears associated with the cost of a nursing home stay. Spell out clearly and in detail exactly what Medicare and Medicaid pay for, and help the patients qualify for these programs. Establishing one's eligibility for Medicaid can be a nightmare, and anything you can do to ease the way will be greatly appreciated. Make sure that private paying patients and their families understand that the rates you quote include or do not include ancillary charges. Do everything you can to avoid misunderstandings over money.

Nursing homes can do much to reduce the uncertainty associated with nursing home placement by having the home's social worker and physical therapist visit the patients in their home. This will help to give you some idea of the individuals' needs and will give the patients a chance to see visible signs of your concern for their welfare. You may even want to arrange for prospective residents to spend a few days in your facility. This trial arrangement will be further evidence to patients that you care about them and that they need not fear poor care and abuse in your home. The fear of being old and ill can be eased by introducing patients to "success stories," that is, to other patients in your home with similar problems who are functioning well.

Do not mix sane, physically infirm patients with the severely mentally retarded or impaired. If you have a high percentage of such patients, realize that you have special problems which will require a larger staff with a great deal of special training. Look to your state department of mental health for the assistance you need, either providing you with trained personnel or in helping you train your own people. You will also want to institute instruction in "death with dignity" to sensitize your employees so that they and the patients they serve can be better able to cope with death.

Finally, do everything you can to preserve the residents' sense of freedom and identity. Give them as many choices as you can possibly arrange. Within the applicable fire codes, allow them to bring to the home their clothes, photographs, favorite chairs, and all the other benchmarks of a lifetime. Do everything possible to protect these valuables from being misplaced or stolen. A tin-type of a beautiful Gibson girl might not mean much to you or your employees, but it might mean a lot more if it were a picture of you taken 60 years ago. The stack of letters and the gold medal might not mean much unless that were all you had left of a son you loved with all your heart. In short, do everything you can to make life pleasant, challenging, informative, and, most of all, interesting.

Chapter 2
Nursing Home Abuses

The best advice to administrators who do not want to be surprised by a law suit or a citation from their state health department owing to negligence on the part of employees is: Be on the premises; let others do the paperwork; take an active interest in patient care and work closely with your nurses. Do not tolerate the slightest breach of duty. Establish an institutional council; meet with employees regularly to learn their suggestions for improvement and to resolve grievances. Allow all the employees to have direct access to your office. Provide a suggestion box or another means for communicating with you confidentially. Working with your nurses, rate each of your employees as if you were a football talent scout; provide merit increases for those who do good work. Honor one employee a month with a $100 savings bond as a bonus for providing excellent care and services.

There are many difficulties which the administrator faces in trying to weed out applicants who have sadistic tendencies. It is almost impossible to tell from appearances which prospective employee will assault your patients. However, you should check each applicant's references and ascertain if s/he has a criminal record or a history of drug abuse. You may still want to hire the person who makes a good impression, even in the face of a minor criminal conviction. However, you naturally want to be alert and monitor the new employee's behavior on the job. You should discipline employees at the first sign that they have physically (or verbally) abused patients. Under the law, both they and you are liable for their acts (both civilly and criminally). As Aspen Systems' *Nursing Home Law Manual* points out, few administrators understand that they may be held accountable for false imprisonment. It cites the case of *Big Town Nursing Home v. Newman*, 461 S.W.2d 195, concerning a patient who was admitted under an agreement that he "would not be forced to remain against his will." When the patient attempted to leave, he was prevented from doing so. He had tried to escape on five or six occasions. Each time he was caught and returned to the home. The patient was sometimes locked and taped in a restraint chair for as long as five hours although there was no evidence that the patient's mental or physical condition warranted restraining devices. The nursing home was found guilty of falsely imprisoning the patient by restraining him without legal justification.

The principal reason for unsanitary conditions is employee indolence or lack of sensitivity. It is up to you to keep your employees working. You may want to dramatize the importance of certain nursing home regulations relating to sanitation. You might use the Baltimore salmonella epidemic as a case history to explain to employees the importance of (a) not letting prepared food sit uncovered at room temperature, (b) not dragging linen through the kitchen, or (c) washing hands after caring for patients. The consequences of an uncontrolled staph infection should also be highlighted. Finally, you should emphasize that few things are more destructive to morale and human dignity than being forced to live in unsanitary conditions when you can do nothing about it.

The key to providing good food in a nursing home is to allow a decent amount in the budget for purchases and a good chef. This means you may have to compete for culinary talent and spend more money for kitchen services, but the results will be worth it. Meals are the one great event that patients have to look forward to. If the meals are poor or even so-so, it sets the tone for the entire operation of the home. You show your staff, your patients and their families how much you care about old people by the meals you serve. Make every effort to have food served when it is warm. The details make all the difference. For your own protection, you will want to lock your walk-in refrigerator and your freezer. Keys should only be given to a few select individuals. Hold them accountable for any shortages.

Remember that you are a trustee of funds given to you by patients and their families. This includes the $25 a month personal spending allowance paid to Medicaid patients. You are liable for any diversion of these funds to your own use. Keep such funds inviolate. Keep meticulous records of any payments made. If interest is earned, make sure it is allocated to the patient's account. When a patient leaves your home, or dies, make sure you have a financial accounting and return to them or their guardians any amounts you have been holding in trust. Do not attempt to keep such funds on the pretext (perhaps justifiable in some states) that Medicaid rates are too low and do not allow you to recover the full cost of providing ancillary services. You may face civil or criminal liability. Make sure patients have their clothing, glasses, etc. marked and returned to them following cleaning or when they are lost. Maintain an inventory of each patient's expensive belongings such as television sets, radios, watches, and jewelry. Designate some personnel as security officers. If any of the patients' possessions disappear, make every effort to have the property returned. Make it clear that you will not tolerate larceny in your home; remind all employees that taking these goods is a crime. If stealing persists, call in the police. You must make it clear early on that stealing is against the home's policy and that violators will be dealt with severely.

Eliminating hazards in nursing homes is a matter of common sense. Most state and federal inspections do a good job of highlighting potential hazards in your physical plant. Make sure you immediately make the corrections which your inspector suggests. As an extra precaution, why not appoint a safety patrol? Once a month have this group conduct a safety check of your entire home from your appliances right down to the food preparation and the quality of patient care. Look for bare wires or shorts in electrical appliances. Check for signs of staph or other infectious diseases. This critical inventory of your facility's safety conducted by employees familiar with your home will give you all the warning you need to institute repairs to protect patients and to avoid unfavorable citations from the department of health.

As noted, the use of restraints should be the absolute last resort. You should take meticulous care that no one is restrained without a specific prescription in writing by a physician, who states the reasons for such confinement and the duration of it. Remember, it's your responsibility to ensure that patients in restraints do not injure themselves. This often means that a patient in restraints requires more time and attention than a patient who is left free. Remind your staff of what can happen. In May of 1976, a 91-year-old woman in a Washington, D.C. nursing home died when the straps used to bind her to the chair cut off her breathing and blood flow.

The best way to avoid being surprised by a complaint triggering an unannounced inspection from the health department is to communicate with your employees, patients, and their families. Establish a cool line — a telephone number that relatives can call to provide complaints anonymously. A locked suggestion box may serve the same purpose. Protect and reward employees who bring you the truth — even if it is unpleasant. Be aggressive in taking action against whatever abuses you find.

The lack of eye care, dental care, and podiatry is a problem in most homes. Aides can provide much of the basic mouth and routine foot care. You probably can make arrangements with local medical and dental societies for the more professional, sophisticated help you need. It is common for them to provide podiatry or dental services free of charge to patients in nursing homes. The same can be said for eye care; call your optometric society. Make a point of having each new patient's eyes examined. In many states, the Medicaid program covers eye care and dental care, so there is little excuse for the elderly, whose care is covered under this program, not to receive the services they need.

Respect for human dignity is the hargest discipline to teach. You must attempt to instill the ideal of the Golden Rule along with a fundamental respect for the intrinsic worth of each individual human being. Try instituting a sensitivity training program. Require each new employee to play the role of a patient for 24 hours prior to hiring them. Have other aides wheel them around dressed only in the familiar hospital gown, give them a bath, place them in restraints for a period of time, feed them, and put them to bed early. Treat them just like all the other patients in the home. This experience will do much to sensitize them to the needs and feelings of patients. It will help them relate to those they care for. More details are in Chapter 14.

Chapter 3
Nursing Home Drugs: Pharmaceutical Russian Roulette

The secret to fewer drug-related abuses in nursing homes is accountability. Limit the access to your medications room. Keep it locked and give out few keys. Hold these people responsible by virtue of pill counts and the like. Be especially careful with narcotics, which must be kept under double lock by federal law. Have your consultant pharmacist help you monitor the use of drugs. Look for any shortages of so-called "uppers" and "downers" such as Elavil and Valium, which have great street value. Your pharmacist can help your nurses watch out for improper combinations of drugs that might affect patients adversely. Remember, the more RNs you use in distributing medications, the fewer errors you will have. Avoid the use of unlicensed personnel for this purpose. Both they and you are liable for mistakes which result in injury, death, or disability. Limit the practice of prescribing drugs over the telephone to emergency situations. Insist on timely visits from physicians to check drug regimens. Consider the installation of unit-dose distribution systems. It will cost you more initially but you will save in two ways: you will free nurses, who would otherwise have the responsibility for setting up and passing drugs, to provide care, and you will eliminate many drug errors. Obviously, the patients will benefit from both developments.

Chapter 4
Nursing Home Fires: A Chronic Condition

Most nursing home patients are old and ill; they are incapable of taking action to save their own lives in case of a major fire. In fact, it may be very difficult to get them to abandon their rooms. Paradoxically, some patients once saved have actually tried to run back into burning buildings. Accordingly, you bear a heavy burden to see that these individuals are protected from fire.

The best protection is, of course, a good fire resistant construction. But even a nursing home made completely out of concrete will burn if it is filled with flammable furnishings such as curtains, nightstands, and the like. Give careful attention to such purchases. Be particularly skeptical of plastic wastebaskets, curtains, vinyl-covered chairs, and cushions stuffed with urethane-like material. Make sure the carpeting you buy has low flammability and smoke generation scores.

Keep your home clean. Do not allow old newspapers or clothes to accumulate in storage areas. Make sure that your electrical wiring is in good condition and prohibit the use of multiple-plug extension cords which may throw an overload on your electrical system. Check your furnace, washing machine, and dryer to see that they are in good working order.

Prohibit smoking in patients' rooms unless there is close supervision by one of your employees or a family member. Provide protected smoking areas where patients, employees, and visitors can smoke. Train your employees in fire prevention and fire fighting techniques. Your local fire department will be glad to help. Numerous lives could have been saved in nursing homes if the staff members had only the presence of mind to close the door to the fire room after attempting to evacuate the patients in it.

While a well-trained staff can reduce the loss of life, it is illogical to expect them to evacuate every patient in your home in case of fire. Smoke and flames travel too quickly to permit this. Automatic heat and smoke detectors are a good first-line protection, but they are not a panacea. In the final analysis, you must train your staff, provide automatic detection devices, *and* install a sprinkling system. This combination will help ensure that your home is not listed in newspapers next winter as the site of a nursing home fire.

Chapter 5
Profiteering: Services to the Needy by the Greedy

The best advice in this area is: Don't yield to temptation and don't be greedy. There may be little in the way of audits to verify the costs you present to Medicare and Medicaid as of this moment, but you can expect intensified interest in these financial statements in the near future. Make every effort to protect the integrity of patients' funds. Forsake asking for kickbacks from your suppliers even though "everybody does it." When you are charged with fraud, it will do you little good to plead (as one operator did) that kickbacks are a common industry practice. Provide families with a clear statement of what they can expect by way of charges.

Resist the temptation to ask the family to subsidize your costs over and above the Medicaid rate or to require them to make a donation as a precondition of admitting them to your facility. This practice is against the law.

Do not blackmail your governor and state legislature with the threat that you will refuse to take Medicaid patients or that you will discharge patients into the street if public assistance rates are not raised. This only serves to perpetuate the money-hungry, ruthless image that some people associate with nursing homes. The most effective way to prove that rates are inadequate is to open your books so that all can see how you are using public funds and to judge for themselves.

Chapter 6
Nursing Homes: New Depositories for the Mentally Impaired

Some 50 to 80 percent of the patients in today's long term care facilities suffer from some degree of mental impairment. But this problem is almost never dealt with in nursing homes, which concentrate on physical illness. Why not obtain a psychiatric evaluation of each patient in addition to the physical examination you provide at the time of admission. This will help you plan an appropriate therapeutic program.

Be wary of mass transfers into your facility from state mental hospitals. Former inmates may fill your empty beds, but they will also increase the burden on your nursing staff. Few of your employees will have had the training to cope with the severely impaired, and you will be hard pressed to carry out the therapeutic program which you would like to offer to all patients. Moreover, there may be sharp increases in mortality and morbidity associated with such transfers. There are some who will attribute these deaths to poor care in your facility rather than to transfer shock.

Again, do not mix the mentally impaired with the sane but physically infirm. The effect can be disastrous to both. Be especially careful in the management of medications. The large doses of potent tranquilizers taken by such patients can result in severe (and often irreversible) side effects. Take special precautions to prevent fire, especially if your impaired aged are ambulatory. Lock flammable liquids away and restrict the availability of matches. If you do have more than a few such patients, call upon your state mental hospital for periodic follow-up evaluations to insure that appropriate psychiatric services are being provided.

Make a lively effort to improve the mental functioning of the infirm aged. Remember Karl Menninger's example of the progress that can be made with even the most hopeless and helpless aged. Educate your staff to the fact that senility and mental impairment in the aged are often reversible with the right kind of effort.

Chapter 7
No Vacancy for Minority Groups

If you are about to build a nursing home, consider an area where ethnic and racial minorities live. The chances are that there will be no nursing home here. You will thus easily qualify for your certificate of need. Logically, there will be a high demand for your services. Most of the residents will qualify for Medicaid, so you will have a ready income, which should provide sufficient collateral for a construction loan from a bank.

You will also have a wealth of potential employees. With a modest amount of training, you will have an excellent staff. These employees will help you relate to the minority aged and vice-versa.

For instant success, make an effort to speak the languages and to understand the customs of the minorities you serve. Bilingual personnel can help the minority aged through the maze of Medicare and Medicaid forms. Try to prepare meals which reflect what these people enjoy at home.

Do everything possible to encourage communication between your facility and the outside community. Let one of your recreation rooms be used for community meetings. Participate in a community meals-on-wheels program. Remember that years of oppression may have left minority groups distrustful of your motives at first. You must earn their trust. In time, it will be clear that you are providing a needed community service and not just another business. Remember also that Title VI of the Civil Rights Act of 1964 prohibits discrimination against any person on account of race, color, or national origin in programs funded by the federal government.

Chapter 9
Lack of a Policy Toward the Infirm Aged

All too often, nursing home providers are perceived as being preoccupied with self-interest. These care-givers could do much for their image by lobbying in their states and in Washington for expanded home health programs which would keep senior citizens independent. Operators need not fear that they will be putting themselves out of business. Most experts in this field concede that there will always be a need for nursing homes and the intensive therapeutic milieu they provide.

For this approach to bolster the stock of providers, the effort must be sincere. It must not be viewed as an attempt by operators to expand their for-profit dealings into the realm of home health services.

Nursing homes should also work to persuade Congress and state legislatures to establish payment formulas which reward good care. One of the best ways to provide credibility is for nursing homes to make their CPA-audited cost and financial statements available to the public. Unfortunately, in the past, operators have been willing to assert they were going broke, but not willing to show their books and records. This cannot help but leave a credibility gap in the minds of policy-makers.

Chapter 10
Enforcement of Standards: A National Farce

The best answer to straightening out nursing home inspections for the operator is to make them unnecessary. One way to do this is with an effective peer review program. If such "self-policing" is instituted, it must be like Caesar's wife — beyond reproach — and must not be taken as another public relations gimmick adopted to save the face of a much-criticized industry. If nursing homes do not comply with standards over a protracted period of time, they should be expelled from state associations. This should be done publically and openly so that it comes to the attention of the news media.

For the present, why not invite unannounced inspections by the press, friends, or families any time, day or night. If you issue such an invitation, then you must be equal to the test. It will mean keeping your home "inspection sharp" all day, every day.

Don't tempt your surveyors with meals, gratuities, or other offers. Their job is hard enough as it is. What you can do is insist that inspectors in your state have the requisite minimum training, education, and experience to do the work they do. If you are cited for deficiencies, make corrections immediately. Never allow the same deficiency to appear in two successive inspection reports. Remember that these reports are public information and that everyone will know what problems you have and how long you have had them.

At the same time, you might encourage your state health department, your county and city health departments, and other agencies to consolidate nursing home inspections. This will save paper as well as wear and tear on you, your staff, and the patients.

Chapter 11
Political Influence and the Nursing Home

There is nothing wrong with contributing funds to the candidate of your choice in an election. The problems in this area generally arise when nursing homes attempt to avoid regulation or to obtain other preferences (such as in obtaining a certificate of need or appointment to a regulatory board) by pulling political strings. An exchange of dollars for political favors is outside the law. Participation in this type of arrangement may put you and your politician both in jail. If you have red tape that needs cutting, hire a lawyer—an independent firm, not one that is affiliated with a prominent politician. Remember that nursing home operators will increasingly live in a fishbowl with the ever-increasing commitment of public funds for the care of the aged.

Chapter 12
The Physician's Abdication of Responsibility

In order to provide adequate medical care for your patients, it is necessary to find a medical director with interest in the aged, who will agree to "ride herd" on individual doctors who have only one or two patients in your home. Physicians need to be reminded of the importance of visiting patients in long term care facilities at scheduled intervals. Make sure that every patient admitted to your home has a physical examination and that patient care plans are established and implemented.

Make arrangements with a second physician who will agree to be on call in the absence of the medical director. Your facility should always have prompt physician coverage in case of an emergency. Establish meaningful transfer agreements with your local hospital and provide for an exchange of personnel. They should understand your operation and you should know theirs as well.

Designate and train a team of nurses to work with the physicians who serve your home. The doctors should be given all the support possible; do everything you can to save their valuable time.

Contact your local medical school and ask if they would be interested in a cooperative agreement whereby their students spend time working and studying in your home.

Chapter 13
Nursing Homes without Nurses

Good care in a nursing home not only involves the services of physicians, but is greatly dependent upon the quality of assistance provided by nurses. The best advice that can be given in this area is: Spend a little more money and hire a few more registered nurses. Generally speaking, the higher the ratio of your RNs to your total population in the home, the better the quality of care. While you're at it, have someone else fill out the Medicare and Medicaid forms. Insist that your RNs distribute medications and that they give patients the direct care which only they are trained to give.

When you get good people, keep them at all costs. You've got to build a team with morale. Your team needs a leader. To keep good people you will have to pay wages that are competitive with what is paid at hospitals. With cost-related reimbursement in effect as of 1978, you should be able to pay adequate salaries and fringe benefits.

Contact your local school of nursing and offer your home as a site for students to study and work with the aged. In return, perhaps they will help you establish a model in-service training program for aides and orderlies and help you establish a career ladder. With appropriate training, education, and experience it should be possible for aides in your facility to work their way up to LPNs, and with further study and experience, finally become full-fledged RNs. You might consider establishing a scholarship program to make this climb a little easier for the financially disadvantaged.

Chapters 14 and 15
America's Finest Nursing Homes
How to Choose a Nursing Home

These chapters describe in detail what consumers will be looking for in a good nursing home and what you might do to make your home one of the best in the nation. When dealing with people looking at nursing homes for their loved ones, the cardinal rule is: Be as honest, open, and helpful as you possibly can. Remember, the family is undergoing a great deal of strain. Be as comforting as you can.

The standout ingredient of a good home is esprit de corps, a basic belief in the worth and dignity of the individual. Other factors include new techniques in rehabilitation, architectural design which improves the delivery and quality of care, new techniques in employee training, and community service. All of these ideas are discussed in detail in Chapter 14.

Chapter 16
Suggestions for Improvement

Many of the suggested reforms in this chapter have already been endorsed by the American Health Care Association, the organization that represents most proprietary facilities. Undoubtedly, you will have little difficulty in agreeing that there should be federal assistance to help train nursing home aides and orderlies or that nursing home benefits should be expanded.

While these proposals have caught the attention of industry policy-makers, nursing home administrators should push just as hard for the expansion of home health programs to keep seniors in their own homes where they most want to be. It would be equally refreshing if nursing home representatives would speak out in favor of more controversial proposals which would increase nursing home standards.

One critical bill would require that registered nurses serve in Medicare and Medicaid nursing homes 24 hours a day. Another would require minimum ratios of nurses to patients. Both of these measures have been vehemently opposed by the industry even though many states have higher standards of their own that are in effect. Another proposal, which has been opposed in some quarters, would increase the fiscal integrity of the Medicare and Medicaid programs by requiring nursing homes to file CPA-audited financial statements. Yet another would allow nursing home patients to bring class action suits against homes which violate standards and provide poor care.

Even though these measures would work against the specific interest of some facilities which are violating the law or providing poor care, they should be supported by most nursing homes in the name of the public good. By lending your support through letters to your elected representatives, you can demonstrate that your interest in human welfare comes before your interest in your own financial welfare.

Appendix C
Where to Turn for Help

The following pages contain several lists of names, addresses and telephone numbers which may be of assistance to those who need to find a nursing home or who have complaints about one. The list includes directors of state health departments, state welfare directors, state attorneys general, state nursing home ombudsmen, key people in the Department of Health, Education, and Welfare, major senior citizens organizations, nursing home action groups and key congressional contacts.

STATE HEALTH DEPARTMENT DIRECTORS

Your state health department licenses and inspects nursing homes for compliance with state and *federal* standards. Complaints to any of the directors listed below with a carbon copy to your congressman will generally bring results.

Alabama
Ira L. Myers, Health Officer
Department of Public Health
State Office Bldg.
501 Dexter Avenue
Montgomery, Alabama 36130
(205) 832-3120

Alaska
Dr. Robert Fraser
Division of Public Health

Department of Health and Social
  Services
503 Alaska Office Bldg.
Juneau, Alaska 99811
(907) 465-3090

Arizona
Suzanne Dandoy, Director
Department of Health Services
1740 W. Adams Street

Phoenix, Arizona 85007
(602) 271-3113

Arkansas
Rex C. Ramsay, Jr., Director
Department of Health
4815 W. Markham Street
Little Rock, Arkansas 72201
(501) 661-2111

California
Jerome A. Lackner, Director
Department of Health
State Office Bldg. 8
714 P Street
Sacramento, California 95814
(916) 445-1248

Colorado
Edward G. Dreyfus, Executive
 Director
Department of Health
4210 E. 11th Avenue
Denver, Colorado 80220
(303) 388-6111, Ext. 315

Connecticut
Douglas S. Lloyd, Commissioner
Department of Health
79 Elm Street
Hartford, Connecticut 06115
(203) 566-2279

Delaware
Barbara B. Rose, M.D., Acting
 Director
Division of Public Health
Department of Health and Social
 Services
Dover, Delaware 19901
(302) 678-4701

District of Columbia
William J. Washington, Jr.,
 Acting Administrator
Community Health and Hospitals
 Administration
Department of Human Resources
1875 Connecticut Avenue, N.W.
Washington, D.C. 20009
(202) 629-3366

Florida
E. Charlton Prather, Staff
 Director
Health Program Office
Department of Health and
 Rehabilitative Services
1323 Winewood Boulevard
Tallahassee, Florida 32301
(904) 488-4115

Georgia
James W. Alley, Director
Division of Physical Health
Department of Human Resources
522 Health Bldg.
47 Trinity Avenue, S.W.
Atlanta, Georgia 30334
(404) 656-4655

Hawaii
George A.L. Yuen, Director
Department of Health
1250 Punchbowl Street
Honolulu, Hawaii 96813
(808) 548-6505

Idaho
John T. Ashley, State Health
 Officer
Division of Health
Department of Health and Welfare

State Office Bldg.
700 W. State Street
Boise, Idaho 83720
(203) 384-3401

Illinois

Joyce C. Lashof, Director
Department of Public Health
525 W. Jefferson Street
Springfield, Illinois 62706
(217) 782-4977

Indiana

William T. Paynter, State Health
  Commissioner
Board of Health
425 Health Bldg.
Indianapolis, Indiana 46206
(317) 633-5490

Iowa

Norman L. Pawlewski,
  Commissioner
Department of Health
E. 12th and Walnut Streets
Des Moines, Iowa 50319
(515) 281-5605

Kansas

Dwight F. Metzler, Secretary
Department of Health and
  Environment
Bldg. 740
Topeka, Kansas 66620
(913) 296-3745

Kentucky

William P. McElwain,
  Commissioner
Bureau for Health Services

Department for Human
  Resources
Health Bldg.
275 E. Main Street
Frankfort, Kentucky 40601
(502) 564-3970

Louisiana

William H. Stewart,
  Commissioner and State
  Health Officer
Health and Human Resources
  Administration
State Office Bldg.
150 Riverside Mall
Baton Rouge, Louisiana 70801
(504) 389-5796

Maine

George E. Sullivan, Director
Bureau of Health
Department of Human Services
State House
Augusta, Maine 04333
(207) 289-3201

Maryland

Neil Solomon, Secretary
Department of Health and Mental
  Hygiene
201 W. Preston Street
Baltimore, Maryland 21201
(301) 383-6195

Massachusetts

Jonathan E. Fielding,
  Commissioner
Department of Public Health
600 Washington Street
Boston, Massachusetts 02111
(617) 727-2700

Michigan

Maurice S. Reizen, Director
Department of Public Health
3500 N. Logan Street
Lansing, Michigan 48909
(517) 373-1320

Minnesota

Walter R. Lawson, Secretary
Department of Health
State Board of Health Bldg.
717 Delaware Street, S.E.
Minneapolis, Minnesota 55440
(612) 296-5460

Mississippi

Alton B. Cobb, Secretary
Mississippi State Board of Health
2423 N. State Street
Jackson, Mississippi 39205
(601) 354-6646

Missouri

Herbert R. Domke, Director
Division of Health
Department of Social Services
High Street and Broadway
Jefferson City, Missouri 65101
(314) 751-4330

Montana

Arthur C. Knight, Acting
    Director
Department of Health and
    Environmental Sciences
200 W. F. Cogswell Bldg.
Helena, Montana 59601
(406) 449-2544

Nebraska

Henry D. Smith, Director

Department of Health
Lincoln Bldg., 2nd Fl.
Lincoln, Nebraska 68508
(402) 471-2133

Nevada

John H. Carr, State Health
    Officer
Health Division
Department of Human Resources
Kinkead Bldg.
505 E. King Street
Carson City, Nevada 89710
(702) 885-4540

New Hampshire

Maynard H. Mites, Director
Division of Public Health
Department of Health and
    Welfare
61 S. Spring Street
Concord, New Hampshire 03301
(603) 271-2526

New Jersey

Joanna E. Finley, Commissioner
Department of Health
John Fitch Plaza
Trenton, New Jersey 08625
(609) 292-7837

New Mexico

Michael J. Burkhart, Director
State Health Agency
Department of Health and Social
    Services
725 St. Michaels Drive
P.O. Box 2348
Santa Fe, New Mexico 37503
(505) 327-3201

New York

Robert P. Whalon, Commissioner
Department of Health
Tower Bldg.
Empire State Plaza
Albany, New York 12237
(518) 474-2011

North Carolina

Jacob Koomen, Director
Division of Health Services
Department of Human Resources
225 N. McDowell Street
Raleigh, North Carolina 27602
(919) 829-3416

North Dakota

Willis Van Heuvelen, Executive
   Officer
Department of Health
State Capitol
Bismarck, North Dakota 58505
(701) 224-2371

Ohio

John Ackerman, Director
Department of Health
450 E. Town Street
Columbus, Ohio 42215
(614) 466-2253

Oklahoma

R. LeRoy Carpenter,
   Commissioner of Health
Department of Health
N.E. 10th and Stonewall Streets
Oklahoma City, Oklahoma 73105
(405) 271-4200

Oregon

Keith Putnam, Administrator

Health Division
Department of Human Resources
930 State Office Bldg.
Portland, Oregon 97201
(503) 229-5032

Pennsylvania

Leonard Bachman, Secretary
Department of Health
802 Health and Welfare Bldg.
Harrisburg, Pennsylvania 17120
(717) 787-6426

Rhode Island

Joseph E. Cannon, Director of
   Health
Department of Health
401 State Health Department
   Bldg.
Providence, Rhode Island 02908

South Carolina

Kenneth E. Aycock,
   Commissioner
Department of Health and
   Environmental Control
2600 Bull Street
Columbia, South Carolina 29201
(803) 758-5443

South Dakota

Judith K. Call, Secretary
Department of Health
Pierre, South Dakota 57501
(605) 224-3361

Tennessee

Eugene W. Fowinkle,
   Commissioner
Department of Public Health
436 6th Avenue, N.

Nashville, Tennessee 37219
(615) 741-3111

Texas

Frans L. Duff, Director
Department of Health Resources
1100 W. 49th Street
Austin, Texas 78756
(512) 454-3781

Utah

Lyman J. Olsen, Director of
  Health
Division of Health
Department of Social Services
44 Medical Drive
Salt Lake City, Utah 84113
(801) 533-6111

Vermont

A.M. McBean, Commissioner
Department of Health
60 Main Street
Burlington, Vermont 05401
(802) 862-5701

Virginia

James B. Kenley, Commissioner
Department of Health
109 Governor Street
Richmond, Virginia 23219
(804) 786-3561

Washington

John Beare, Director
Health Services Division
Department of Social and Health
  Services
Olympia, Washington 98504
(206) 753-5871

West Virginia

Newman H. Dyer, Director
Department of Health
535 State Office Bldg. 3
Charleston, West Virginia 25305
(304) 348-2971

Wisconsin

George H. Handy, Health Officer
Division of Health
Department of Health and Social
  Services
434 Wilson Street
State Office Bldg.
Madison, Wisconsin 53701
(608) 266-1511

Wyoming

Harvey Peterson, Coordinator
Department of Health and Social
  Services
2300 Capitol Avenue
Cheyenne, Wyoming 82002
(307) 777-7657

STATE WELFARE DIRECTORS

As a precondition of participating in the Medicaid program, States are required to designate one agency which is responsible for the overall operation of that program. Such designated agencies are called "single state agencies." Most often your local welfare department carries that title. The individuals listed below have responsibility over eligibility for Medicaid in their respective states to insure that the state Medicaid program is free from fraud and abuse and otherwise is being administered properly.

Medicaid
Single State Agencies: Welfare Directors

Alabama

Robert H. Holzworth, M.D.
Director, Medical Services Administration
Alabama Dept. of Public Health
2500 Fairlane Drive
Montgomery, Alabama 36104
(205) 277-2710

Guy L. Burns
Department of Pensions and Security
Administration Building
Montgomery, Alabama 36130
(205) 832-6095

Alaska

Dr. Francis S.L. Williamson
Commissioner, Dept. of Health & Social Service
Pouch H
Juneau, Alaska 99801
(907) 465-3030

Arizona

Gary D. Hulshoff, Ph.D.
Division of Medical Assistance
State Department Bldg.
1740 W. Adams Street
Phoenix, Arizona 85001
(602) 271-3387

John Huerta
Director

Department of Economic Security
Box 6123
Phoenix, Arizona 85005
(602) 271-5678

Arkansas

Mr. James Cartwright
Commissioner
Arkansas Social Services
P. O. Box 1437
Little Rock, Arkansas 72201
(501) 371-2521

David Ray
Director
Department of Social and Rehabilitative Services
401 National Old Line Building
Little Rock, Arkansas 72203
(501) 371-1001

California

Dr. Jerome A. Lackner
Director
Dept. of Health
714 P Street
Office Bldg. No. 8
Sacramento, California 95814
(916) 445-1248

Marion Woods
Director
Department of Benefit Payments

Health and Welfare Agency
744 "P" Street
Sacramento, California 95814
(916) 445-4500

Colorado
Mr. Henry A. Foley
Executive Director
Dept. of Public Welfare
1575 Sherman Street
Denver, Colorado 80203
(303) 892-3515

Connecticut
Mr. Edward W. Maher
Commissioner
Dept. of Social Services
110 Bartholomew Avenue
Hartford, Connecticut 06105
(203) 566-2008

Delaware
Mr. Charles H. Debnam
Acting Secretary
Dept. of Health and Social
   Services
Delaware State Hospital
New Castle, Delaware 19720
(302) 412-6705

District of Columbia
Albert P. Russo
Acting Director
Dept. of Human Resources
District Bldg., Rm. 406
Washington, D.C. 20004
(202) 629-5443

William Bar
Administrator

Social Rehabilitation Administration
122 "C" Street, N.W.
Washington, D.C. 20001
(202) 629-3745

Florida
Mr. O. J. Keller
Secretary
Dept. of Health and
   Rehabilitation Services
1323 Winewood Blvd.
Tallahassee, Florida 32301

Charles Hall
Director
Department of Health and
   Rehabilitative Services
1311 Winewood Boulevard
Jacksonville, Florida 32203
(904) 725-3080

Georgia
Mr. T. M. (Jim) Parham
Acting Commissioner
Georgia Dept. of Human
   Resources
State Office Building
Atlanta, Georgia 30334
(404) 656-4680

Douglas Skelton
Commissioner
Department of Human
   Resources
47 Trinity Avenue, S.W.
Atlanta, Georgia 30334
(404) 656-4414

Hawaii
Mr. Andrew I. T. Chang

Director, Dept. of Social Service
  & Housing
P. O. Box 339
Honolulu, Hawaii 96809
(808) 548-6584

Edwin B.L. Tam
Administrator
Public Welfare Division
Department of Social
  Services and Housing
Queen Liliuokalani Building
Honolulu, Hawaii 96813
(808) 548-5908

Idaho

Mr. Karl E. Banschbach
Director of Medical Assistance
Department of Health and
  Welfare
State House
Boise, Idaho 83720
(208) 964-3556

Milton G. Klein
Director
Department of Health and
  Welfare
700 W. State Street
Boise, Idaho 83720
(208) 384-2336

Illinois

Mr. James Trainor
Director, Dept. of Public Aid
618 E. Washington St.
Springfield, Illinois 62706
(217) 549-6716

Donald H. Schlosser
Acting Director

Department of Children
  and Family Services
Springfield, Illinois 62706
(212) 782-7615

Indiana

Mr. Wayne Stanton
Administrator
Indiana State Dept. of Public
  Welfare
100 N. Senate Ave., Rm. 701
Indianapolis, Indiana 46204
(317) 633-6650

Iowa

Mr. Kevin Burns
Commissioner
Iowa Dept. of Social Service
Lucas State Office Bldg.
Des Moines, Iowa 50319
(515) 281-5452

Kansas

Dr. Robert C. Harder
State Director of Social and
  Rehabilitative Services
10th and Topeka Avenue
State Office Building
Topeka, Kansas 66612
(913) 296-3271

Kentucky

Mr. C. Leslie Dawson
Secretary
Dept. Human Resources
Capitol Annex
Frankfort, Kentucky 40601
(502) 564-3703

Gail S. Huecker
Commissioner

Bureau of Social Insurance
Department of Human
    Resources
New Capitol Annex Room 201
Frankfort, Kentucky 40601
(502) 564-3703

Louisiana

Dr. William H. Stewart
Commissioner
Dept. of Public Welfare
P. O. Box 44065
Baton Rouge, Louisiana 70804
(504) 389-5796

William A. Cherry
Director
Department of Health and
    Human Resources
150 Riverside Mall
Baton Rouge, Louisiana 70802
(504) 389-6036

Maine

Mr. David Smith
Commissioner
Dept. of Human Services
221 State Street
Augusta, Maine 04330
(207) 289-2736

Maryland

Mr. J. C. Eshelman
Director
Division of Medical Care
    Programs Administration
Dept. of Health and Mental
    Hygiene
301 W. Preston Street
Baltimore, Maryland 21201

Richard A. Batterton
Secretary
Department of Human
    Resources
1100 N. Eutaw Street
Baltimore, Maryland 21201
(301) 383-5528

Massachusetts

Mr. Alexander Sharp
Commissioner
Dept. of Public Welfare
600 Washington Street
Boston, Massachusetts 02111
(617) 727-6190

Michigan

Dr. John T. Dempsey
Director, Michigan Dept. of Social
    Services
Commerce Center Building
300 South Capitol Avenue
Lansing, Michigan 48926
(517) 373-2000

Minnesota

Mrs. Vera J. Likins
Commissioner
Dept. of Public Welfare
Centennial Office Bldg.
658 Cedar Street
St. Paul, Minnesota 55155
(612) 296-2701

Mississippi

Mr. Bryan Holliday
Acting Director
Mississippi Medicaid Commission
Room 313, Dale Building
2906 N. State Street

Jackson, Mississippi 39216
(601) 354-7464

Fred W. Sinclair
Commissioner
Public Welfare Department
Box 4321
Jackson, Mississippi 39216

Missouri

James F. Walsh
Director
Department of Social Services
High Street and Broadway
Jefferson City, Missouri 65101
(314) 751-4247

Montana

Patrick E. Melby
Director, Department of Social
   and Rehabilitative Services
P.O. Box 4210
Helena, Montana 59601
(406) 449-3451

Nebraska

Eldin J. Ehrlich
Director
Department of Public Welfare
301 Centennial Mall South
   Fifth Floor
Lincoln, Nebraska 68508
(402) 471-2366

Nevada

Mr. George E. Miller
Administrator, Welfare Division
Dept. of Human Resources
251 Jeanelle Dr.
Carson City, Nevada 89701
(702) 885-4775

New Hampshire

Richard G. Lacombe
Director, Division of Welfare
Department of Health and
   Welfare
8 Loudon Street
Concord, New Hampshire 03301
(603) 271-2286

New Jersey

Ms. Ann Klein
Commissioner
Dept. of Institutions and
   Agencies
135 West Hanover
Trenton, New Jersey 08625

G. Thomas Riti
Director
Division of Public Welfare
Department of Human Services
3525 Quakerbridge Road
Trenton, New Jersey 08618
(609) 890-9500

New Mexico

Mr. Richard W. Heim
Executive Director
New Mexico Health and Social
   Service Dept.
P. O. Box 2348
Santa Fe, New Mexico 87501
(505) 827-2371

Charles Lopez
Administrator
Social Welfare Programs
Health and Social Services
   Department
PERA Building, Room 301

Sante Fe, New Mexico 87501
(505) 827-2371

New York

Philip L. Toia
Commissioner
State Dept. of Social Services
1450 N. Pearl Street
Albany, New York 12243
(518) 457-7051

North Carolina

Robert H. Ward
Division of Social
   Services
Department of Human Resources
Albemarle Building
Raleigh, North Carolina 27611
(919) 733-3055

North Dakota

Mr. T. N. Tangedahl
Executive Director
Social Service Board of North
   Dakota
State Capitol Building
Bismarck, North Dakota 58505
(701) 244-2310

Ohio

Kwegyir Aggrey
Director
Dept. of Public Welfare
30 E. Broad Street
Columbus, Ohio 43215
(614) 466-6282

Oklahoma

Mr. Lloyd E. Rader
Director, Dept. of Institutions
Social and Rehabilitation Service

P. O. Box 25352
Oklahoma City, Oklahoma 73125
(405) 521-3646

Oregon

Linda Kaeser
Administrator
Public Welfare Division
Department of Human Resources
400 Public Service Building
Salem, Oregon 97310
(503) 378-3680

Pennsylvania

Mr. Frank S. Beal
Secretary, State Dept. of Public
   Welfare
333 Health and Welfare Bldg.
Harrisburg, Pennsylvania 17120
(717) 787-2600

Rhode Island

Mr. John J. Affleck
Director, Dept. of Social and
   Rehabilitation Service
Aime J. Forand Bldg.
600 New London Avenue
Cranston, Rhode Island 02920
(401) 464-2121

South Carolina

Robert D. Floyd
Interim Commissioner
Department of Social Services
Box 1520
Columbia, South Carolina 29202
(803) 758-3244

South Dakota

Orval Westby
Secretary

Department of Social Services
State Office Building
Pierre, South Dakota 57501
(605) 224-3491

Tennessee

Eugene W. Fowinkle, M.D.
Commissioner, State Dept. of
   Public Health
344 Cordell Hull Bldg.
Nashville, Tennessee 37219
(615) 741-3666

Horace Bass
Commissioner
Department of Human Services
410 State Office Building
Nashville, Tennessee 37219
(615) 741-3241

Texas

Mr. Raymond W. Vowell
Commissioner, State Dept. of
   Public Welfare
John H. Reagan Bldg.
Austin, Texas 78701
(512) 475-5777

Utah

Mr. Paul S. Rose
Executive Director
Dept. of Social Services
211 State Capitol
Salt Lake City, Utah 84111
(801) 328-5331

Lloyd Nelson
Interim Director
Division of Family Services
Department of Social Services
333 S. 2nd East

Salt Lake City, Utah 84111
(801) 533-5031

Vermont

Mr. Paul R. Philbrook
Commissioner
Dept. of Social Welfare
87 Main Street
Montpelier, Vermont 05602
(802) 828-3421

Virginia

Dr. Mack I. Shanholtz
Commissioner
State Dept. of Health
109 Governor Street
Richmond, Virginia 23219
(804) 770-3561

William L. Luckhard
Commissioner
Department of Welfare
8007 Discovery Drive
Blair Building
Richmond, Virginia 23219
(840) 786-8571

Washington

Harland P. McNutt
Dept. of Social and Health Service
M.S.440
Olympia, Washington 98504
(206) 753-3395

West Virginia

Mrs. Helen Condry
Director, Division of Medical Care
Dept. of Welfare
1900 Washington St., East
Charleston, West Virginia 25305
(304) 345-8990

Leon H. Ginsberg
Commissioner
Department of Welfare
State Office Building 6
Charleston, West Virginia 25305
(304) 348-2400

Wyoming

Lawrence J. Cohen, M.D.
Administrator, Division of Health
    and Medical Services
Dept. of Health and Social Service
State Office Building
Cheyenne, Wyoming 82001
(307) 777-7658

Wisconsin

Manuel Carballo
Secretary
Department of Health and
    Social Service
1 W. Wilson Street
Madison, Wisconsin 53702
(608) 266-3681

Jeremy Wight
Administrator
Division of Public Assistance
    and Social Services
Department of Health and
    Social Services
Hathaway Building
Cheyenne, Wyoming 82002
(307) 777-7561

STATE ATTORNEYS GENERAL

The individuals listed below are the highest law officers in your
state. You may want to turn to them or to your district attorney if you
feel the law has been broken or that a crime has been committed. If you
believe there has been a breach of federal law (including Medicare and
Medicaid fraud), you may wish to contact your local United States
Attorney.

Attorneys General of the States

Alabama

Honorable William J. Baxley
Attorney General of Alabama
State Administration Building
Montgomery, Alabama 36104
(205) 834-5150

Alaska

Honorable Avrum Gross
Attorney General of Alaska

Pouch K, State Capitol
Juneau, Alaska 99801
(907) 465-3600

Arizona

Honorable Bruce Babbitt
Attorney General of Arizona
1700 W. Washington Street
Phoenix, Arizona 85007
(602) 271-4266

Arkansas

Honorable Bill Clinton
Justice Building
Little Rock, Arkansas 72201
(501) 371-2007

California

Honorable Evelle J. Younger
Attorney General of California
555 Capitol Mall
Sacramento, California 95814
(916) 445-4334

Colorado

Honorable John D. MacFarlane
Attorney General of Colorado
104 State Capitol
Denver, Colorado 80203
(303) 892-2541

Connecticut

Honorable Carl R. Ajello
Attorney General of Connecticut
Capitol Annex, 30 Trinity Street
Hartford, Connecticut 06115
(203) 566 2026

Delaware

Honorable Richard R. Wier, Jr.
Attorney General of Delaware
Department of Justice
Wilmington, Delaware 19801
(302) 571-2500

District of Columbia

John R. Risher
Corporation Counsel
D.C. Building
Washington, D.C. 20004
(202) 629-3858

Florida

Honorable Robert L. Shevin
Attorney General of Florida
State Capitol
Tallahassee, Florida 32304
(904) 488-5861

Georgia

Honorable Arthur K. Bolton
Attorney General of Georgia
132 State Judicial Building
Atlanta, Georgia 30334
(404) 656-4586

Hawaii

Honorable Ronald Amemiya
Attorney General of Hawaii
State Capitol
Honolulu, Hawaii 96813
(808) 548-4740

Idaho

Honorable Wayne L. Kidwell
Attorney General of Idaho
State Capitol
Boise, Idaho 83720
(208) 384-2400

Illinois

Honorable William J. Scott
Attorney General of Illinois
500 South Second
Springfield, Illinois 62701
(217) 782-1090

Indiana

Honorable Theodore L. Sendak
Attorney General of Indiana
219 State House
Indianapolis, Indiana 46204
(317) 633-5512

Iowa

Honorable Richard D. Turner
Attorney General of Iowa
State Capitol
Des Moines, Iowa 50319
(515) 281-5164

Kansas

Honorable Curt T. Schneider
Attorney General of Kansas
State House
Topeka, Kansas 66612
(913) 296-2215

Kentucky

Honorable Robert Stephens
Attorney General of Kentucky
State Capitol
Frankfort, Kentucky 40601
(502) 564-7600

Louisiana

Honorable William J. Guste, Jr.
Attorney General of Louisiana
P. O. Box 44005
Baton Rouge, Louisiana 60804
(504) 389-6761

Maine

Honorable Joseph E. Brennan
Attorney General of Maine
State House
Augusta, Maine 04330
(207) 289-3661

Maryland

Honorable Francis B. Burch
Attorney General of Maryland
One South Calvert Street
Baltimore, Maryland 21202
(301) 383-3737

Massachusetts

Honorable Francis X. Bellotti
Attorney General of
   Massachusetts
State House
Boston, Massachusetts 92133
(617) 727-2216

Michigan

Honorable Frank J. Kelley
Attorney General of Michigan
Law Building
Lansing, Michigan 48902
(517) 373-1110

Minnesota

Honorable Warren R. Spannaus
Attorney General of Minnesota
102 State Capitol
St. Paul, Minnesota 55155
(612) 296-2591

Mississippi

Honorable A. F. Summer
Attorney General of Mississippi
State Capitol
Jackson, Mississippi 39205
(601) 354-7130

Missouri

Honorable John Ashcroft
Attorney General of Missouri
Supreme Court Building
Jefferson City, Missouri 65101
(314) 751-3321

Montana

Honorable Mike Greely
Attorney General of Montana
State Capitol

Helena, Montana 59601
(406) 449-2026

Nebraska

Honorable Paul L. Douglas
Attorney General of Nebraska
State Capitol
Lincoln, Nebraska 68509
(402) 471-2682

Nevada

Honorable Robert List
Attorney General of Nevada
Supreme Court Building
Carson City, Nevada 89701
(702) 885-4170

New Hampshire

Honorable David H. Souter
Attorney General of New
  Hampshire
State House Annex
Concord, New Hampshire 03301
(603) 271-3655

New Jersey

Honorable William F. Hyland
Attorney General of New Jersey
State House Annex
Trenton, New Jersey 08625
(609) 292-4925

New Mexico

Honorable Toney Anaya
Attorney General of New Mexico
Supreme Court Building
  P.O. Box 2246
Santa Fe, New Mexico 87501
(505) 827-2844

New York

Honorable Louis J. Lefkowitz
Attorney General of New York
State Capitol
Albany, New York 12224
(518) 474-7330

North Carolina

Honorable Rufus L. Edmisten
Attorney General of North
  Carolina
Justice Building, P. O. Box 629
Raleigh, North Carolina 27602
(919) 829-3377

North Dakota

Honorable Allen I. Olson
Attorney General of North
  Dakota
State Capitol
Bismarck, North Dakota 58501
(701) 224-2210

Ohio

Honorable William J. Brown
Attorney General of Ohio
State House Annex
Columbus, Ohio 43215
(614) 466-3376

Oklahoma

Honorable Larry Derryberry
Attorney General of Oklahoma
112 State Capitol
Oklahoma City, Oklahoma 73105

Oregon

Honorable R. Lee Johnson
Attorney General of Oregon
100 State Office Building
Salem, Oregon 97310

Pennsylvania

Honorable Robert P. Kane
Attorney General of
    Pennsylvania
Capitol Annex, Room 1
Harrisburg, Pennsylvania 17120
(717) 787-3391

Rhode Island

Honorable Julius C. Michaelson
Attorney General of Rhode Island
Providence County Courthouse
Providence, Rhode Island 02903
(401) 831-6850

South Carolina

Honorable Daniel R. McLeod
Attorney General of South
    Carolina
Hampton Office Building
Columbia, South Carolina 29201
(803) 758-3970

South Dakota

Honorable William Janklow
Attorney General of South
    Dakota
State Capitol
Pierre, South Dakota 57501
(605) 224-3215

Tennessee

Honorable R. A. Ashley, Jr.
Attorney General of Tennessee
Supreme Court Building
Nashville, Tennessee 37219
(615) 741-3491

Texas

Honorable John L. Hill
Attorney General of Texas
Supreme Court Building
    Box 12548
Austin, Texas 78711
(512) 475-4643

Utah

Honorable Robert Hansen
Attorney General of Utah
State Capitol
Salt Lake City, Utah 84114
(801) 533-5261

Vermont

Honorable M. Jerome Diamond
Attorney General of Vermont
Pavilion Office Building
Montpelier, Vermont 05602
(802) 828-3171

Virginia

Honorable Andrew P. Miller
Attorney General of Virginia
Supreme Court — Library
    Building
Richmond, Virginia 23219
(804) 786-2071

Washington

Honorable Slade Gorton
Attorney General of Washington
Temple of Justice
Olympia, Washington 98504
(206) 753-2550

West Virginia

Honorable Chauncey H.
    Browning, Jr.
Attorney General of West
    Virginia
State Capitol

Charleston, West Virginia 25304
(304) 348-2021

Madison, Wisconsin 53702
(608) 266-1221

Wyoming

Honorable V. Frank Mendicino

Wisconsin

Attorney General of Wyoming

Honorable Bronson C. LaFollette

210 State Capitol

Attorney General of Wisconsin

Cheyenne, Wyoming 82001

Department of Justice

(307) 777-7841

   114E State Capitol

STATE NURSING HOME OMBUDSMEN

Under pressure from Senators Moss and Percy, HEW established several model nursing home ombudsman projects. An ombudsman is a patients' advocate. It is his or her job to help resolve nursing home complaints. Beginning in 1976, HEW, through the Administration on Aging, made funds available to all the states to establish such units. A list of these officers follows.

Nursing Home Ombudsman Program

CENTRAL OFFICE

Willis Atwell, Acting Director
Sue Wheaton, Program Analyst
Denise Shipp, Secretary
Nursing Home Interests Staff
Administration on Aging
330 Independence Avenue, S.W.
Room 4746 - HEW North Bldg.
Washington, D.C. 20201
(202) 245-6810

REGION I

George Molloy
Regional Liaison
Nursing Home Ombudsman
   Program
Office of Aging, DHEW Region I
John Fitzgerald Kennedy Bldg.
Room 200
Boston, Massachusetts 02203
(617) 223-6885

Connecticut

Jacqueline Walker
Nursing Home Ombudsman
   Program
Connecticut Department on
   Aging
90 Washington Street
Hartford, Connecticut 06115
(203) 566-2480 X29

Maine

Richard Michaud, Director
Bureau of Maine's Elderly
Department of Human Services
State House
Augusta, Maine 04333
(207) 289-2561

Trish Riley, Director
Susan Young

Nursing Home Ombudsman
  Program
Maine Committee on Aging
State House
Augusta, Maine 04333
(207) 289-2561

Massachusetts

John J. Donovan, Director
Massachusetts Nursing Home
  Ombudsman Program
Office of Elder Affairs
120 Boylston Street
Boston, Massachusetts 02116
(617) 727-7273

New Hampshire

Charles Hitchcock
Nursing Home Ombudsman
  Program
New Hampshire State Council on
  Aging
14 Depot Street (P.O. Box 786)
Concord, New Hampshire 03301
(603) 271-2751

Rhode Island

Joseph R. Marocco
Nursing Home Ombudsman
  Program
Division on Aging
150 Washington Street
Providence, Rhode Island 02908
(401) 277-2858

Vermont

Gwen McGrath
Nursing Home Ombudsman
  Program
Office on Aging
81 River Street

Montpelier, Vermont 05602
(802) 828-2751

REGION II

Arthur Wolfe
Regional Liaison
Nursing Home Ombudsman
  Program
Office of Aging, DHEW Region II
26 Federal Plaza, Room 4106
New York, New York 10007
(212) 264-4592

New Jersey

John Walzer
Nursing Home Ombudsman
  Program
Office of Human Resources—
Legal Services
Department of Community
  Affairs
363 West State Street
Trenton, New Jersey 08625
(609) 292-8658

New York

Karen Comeaux
Nursing Home Ombudsman
  Program
New York State Office on Aging
Agency Bldg. #2, Empire State
  Plaza
Albany, New York
(518) 474-5796

Puerto Rico

Lourves Machargo
Nursing Home Ombudsman
  Program

Puerto Rico Gericulture
  Commission
Hawayek Building, Stop 18
Santurce, Puerto Rico
(809) 723-9432 or 725-8015

REGION III
Allen Tyson
Regional Liaison
Nursing Home Ombudsman
  Program
Office of Aging, DHEW Region
  III
P.O. Box 13716 (3535 Market St.)
Philadelphia, Pennsylvania 19101
(215) 596-6891

Delaware
Elizabeth Pattison
Nursing Home Ombudsman
  Program
Division of Aging
2413 Lancaster Avenue
Wilmington, Delaware 19805
(302) 571-3481

District of Columbia
Karyn Barquin
Nursing Home Ombudsman
  Program
Services to the Aged
1329 E Street, N.W.
Washington, D.C. 20004
(202) 638-2406

Maryland
Dr. Matthew Tayback
Director, Office on Aging
State Office Building
301 West Preston Street

Baltimore, Maryland 21201
(301) 383-5064

Dorothy S. Doyle
Nursing Home Ombudsman
  Program
Maryland Office on Aging
State Office Building
301 West Preston Street
Baltimore, Maryland 21201
(301) 383-5064

Pennsylvania
Donna McDowell
Coordinator
Long Term Care Advocacy
  Program
Office for the Aging
Health and Welfare Bldg.
  Room 506
Harrisburg, Pennsylvania 17120
(717) 783-1849

Carol A. Delany
Director, Pennsylvania Nursing
  Home Ombudsman Project
133 South 36th, Room 501
Philadelphia, Pennsylvania 19104
(215) 238-7776

Virginia
Kathleen Fisher
Nursing Home Ombudsman
  Program
Virginia Office on Aging
830 E. Main Street, Suite 950
Richmond, Virginia 23219
(804) 786-7894

West Virginia
Ann Stottlemeyer
Nursing Home Ombudsman
  Program

West Virginia Commission on
Aging
State Capitol
Charleston, West Virginia 25305
(304) 348-2243

REGION IV
Thelma Langley
Regional Liaison
Nursing Home Ombudsman
Program
Office of Aging, DHEW Region IV
50 Seventh St., N.E., Rm. 326
Atlanta, Georgia 30323
(404) 881-2042

Alabama

Price Stone
Nursing Home Ombudsman
Program
Alabama Commission on Aging
740 Madison Avenue
Montgomery, Alabama 36130
(205) 832-6640

Georgia

Faith Ponder
Nursing Home Ombudsman
Program
Georgia Office on Aging
618 Ponce DeLeon Avenue, N.E.
Atlanta, Georgia 30308
(404) 894-5341

Florida

Beth Sodeck
Nursing Home Ombudsman
Program
Office of Aging and Adult
Services

Dept. of Health & Rehabilitative
Services
1323 Winewood Boulevard,
Rm. 425
Tallahassee, Florida 32301
(904) 487-1681

Kentucky

Harold Mann
Aging Branch
Bureau of Aging Services
403 Wapping Street
Bush Building
Frankfort, Kentucky 40601
(502) 564-6930

Betty Gillispie
Nursing Home Ombudsman
Program
Department of Human Resources
316 Wilkinson
Frankfort, Kentucky 40601
(502) 564-5497

Mississippi

Bill Jordan
Nursing Home Ombudsman
Program
Mississippi Council on Aging
P.O. Box 5136, Fondren Station
510 George Street
Jackson, Mississippi 39216
(601) 354-6590

North Carolina

Robert Q. Beard
Executive Director
Office for Aging
Department of Human Resources
213 Hillsborough Street
Raleigh, North Carolina 27603
(919) 829-3983

Edward D. Champion
Nursing Home Ombudsman
    Program
Office on Aging
213 Hillsborough Street
Raleigh, North Carolina 27603
(919) 733-3983

South Carolina

Bill Bradley, Director
Nursing Home Ombudsman
    Program
South Carolina Commission on
    Aging
915 Main Street
Columbia, South Carolina 29201
(803) 758-2576

Tennessee

William M. Stephens
Nursing Home Ombudsman
    Program
Tennessee Commission on Aging
S and P Building, Suite 102
306 Gay Street
Nashville, Tennessee
(615) 741 3056

Melissa Jones
Tennessee-Virginia Development
    District Nursing Home
    Ombudsman
201½ Perry Street
Elizabethton, Tennessee 37643

Edna Foster
Southeast Tennessee Nursing
    Home Ombudsman Program
2501 Milne Avenue
Chattanooga, Tennessee 37406

REGION V
William Watt

Regional Liaison
Nursing Home Ombudsman
    Program
Office of Aging, DHEW Region V
300 South Wacker Drive, 15th Fl.
Chicago, Illinois 60606
(312) 353-4695

Illinois

George L. Stanton
Nursing Home Ombudsman
    Program
Illinois Department on Aging
2401 West Jefferson Street
Springfield, Illinois 62706
(217) 783-5773

Indiana

Sherry Simons
Nursing Home Ombudsman
    Program
Indiana Commission on Aging and
    Aged
Graphic Arts Building
215 North Senate Avenue
Indianapolis, Indiana 46202
(317) 633-5948

Michigan

Ron Kivi
Acting Director
Office of Services to the Aging
3500 North Logan Street
Lansing, Michigan 48913
(517) 373-8230

Doug Roberts, Director
Citizens for Better Care
Nursing Home Ombudsman
    Program
855 Grove

East Lansing, Michigan 48823
(517) 337-1676

Minnesota

Diane Justice
Director of Planning and Policy
 Analysis
Governor's Citizens Council on
 Aging
Suite 204 Metro Square Building
7th and Roberts Streets
St. Paul, Minnesota 55117
(612) 296-2770

Judy Sivak
Nursing Home Ombudsman
 Program
Governor's Citizens Council on
 Aging
Suite 204 Metro Square Building
7th and Roberts Streets
St. Paul, Minnesota 55117
(612) 296-3837

Ohio

Catherine Worley
Nursing Home Ombudsman
 Program
Ohio Commission on Aging
34 North High Street
Columbus, Ohio 43215
(614) 466-5500

Wisconsin

Duane Willadsen, Administrator
Division on Aging
Dept. of Health & Social Services
1 West Wilson Street, Rm. 686
Madison, Wisconsin 53702
(608) 266-2536

David J. Krings
Nursing Home Ombudsman

Program
Office of the Lieutenant Governor
GEF - Room 498
201 East Washington Street
Madison, Wisconsin 53702
(608) 266-8944

Judy Zitske
Nursing Home Ombudsman
 Program
Oneida County Commission on
 Aging
Oneida County Courthouse
Rhinelander, Wisconsin 54501
(715) 369-1505

REGION VI

Anne Bayne
Regional Liaison
Nursing Home Ombudsman
 Program
Office of Aging, DHEW Region VI
1507 Pacific Avenue
Fidelity Union Tower Bldg.,
 Room 50
Dallas, Texas 75201
(214) 749-7286

Arkansas

Erma Petty
Nursing Home Ombudsman
 Program
Office on Aging and Adult
 Services
Dept. of Social and Rehabilitative
 Services
7107 W. 12th Street
Westpark #2 (3rd Floor)
P.O. Box 2179
Little Rock, Arkansas 72203
(501) 371-2441

Louisiana

Janet Slaybaugh
Planning Officer
Bureau of Aging Services
150 Riverside Mall
Baton Rouge, Louisiana 70804
(318) 389-2171

Elaine Bennett
Nursing Home Ombudsman
  Program
Bureau of Aging Services
150 Riverside Mall
Baton Rouge, Louisiana 70804
(318) 389-2171

New Mexico

Marjorie Goetz
Nursing Home Ombudsman
  Program
Commission on Aging
408 Galisteo
Santa Fe, New Mexico 87501
(505) 827-5258

Texas

William R. Thomas
Deputy Director
Governor's Committee on Aging
P.O. Box 12786-Capitol Station
Austin, Texas 78711
(512) 475-2717

Douglas Richnow
Nursing Home Oumbudsman
  Program
Texas Legal Protection Plan
Texas Bar Association
P.O. Box 12487
Austin, Texas 78711
(512) 476-6823
WATS:(800) 492-4141

REGION VII

Lila Waldrop
Regional Liaison
Nursing Home Ombudsman
  Program
Office of Aging, DHEW Region
  VII
601 E. 12th Street
Kansas City, Missouri 64106
(816) 374-2955

Kansas

Edgerton Taylor
Nursing Home Ombudsman
  Program
Services for the Aging
2700 West 6th
Topeka, Kansas 66606
(913) 296-4986

Iowa

Paul Vanderburgh
Nursing Home Ombudsman
  Program
Commission on Aging
415 West 10th Street
Des Moines, Iowa 50319
(515) 281-5187

Nebraska

Nursing Home Ombudsman
  Program
Commission on Aging
State House Station 94784
Lincoln, Nebraska 68509
(402) 471-2307

REGION VIII

Clinton Hess
Director, Office of Aging,
  DHEW — Region VIII

19th & Stout Streets, Rm. 7430
Federal Office Building
Denver, Colorado 80202
(303) 837-2951

Colorado

Phil Nathanson
Division of Services for the Aging
Department of Social Services
1575 Sherman Street
Denver, Colorado 80203
(303) 892-2641/2586

George Hacker
Nursing Home Ombudsman
    Program
Senior Citizens Law Center
912 Broadway
Denver, Colorado 80203
(303) 837-1313

Montana

Rich King
Nursing Home Ombudsman
    Program
Aging Services Bureau
Dept. of Social and Rehabilitation
    Services
P.O. Box 1723
Helena, Montana 59601
(406) 449-3124

North Dakota

Jo Hildebrandt
Nursing Home Ombudsman
    Program
Aging Services
Social Services Board of
    North Dakota
State Capitol Building
Bismarck, North Dakota 58505
(701) 224-2577

South Dakota

Jim Anderson
Director, Office on Aging
Department of Social Services
Kneip Building
Pierre, South Dakota 57501
(605) 224-3656

Barbara McCandless
Katherine H. DeZonia
Nursing Home Ombudsman
    Program
Dept. of Commerce & Consumer
    Affairs
Pierre, South Dakota 57501
(605) 224-3177

Utah

Ronald D. Hampton
Programs Coordinator
Utah State Division on Aging
345 South 6th East
Salt Lake City, Utah 84117
(801) 328-6422

Nursing Home Ombudsman
    Program
Department of Social Services
State Capitol Building, Rm. 104
Salt Lake City, Utah 84114
(801) 533-5331

Wyoming

Nursing Home Ombudsman
    Program
Aging Services
Dept. of Health & Social Services
Division of Public Assistance
New State Office Bldg., West
Room 288
Cheyenne, Wyoming 82002
(307) 777-7561

REGION IX

Dave Coher
Regional Liaison
Nursing Home Ombudsman
  Program
Office of Aging, DHEW Region
  IX
50 United Nations Plaza, Rm. 206
San Francisco, California 94102
(415) 556-2930

Arizona

Gary Anderson
Nursing Home Ombudsman
  Program
Bureau of Aging
Department of Economic Security
P. O. Box 6123
Phoenix, Arizona 85005
(602) 271-4446

California

Loretta Petersen
Nursing Home Ombudsman
  Program
California State Office on Aging
Sacramento, California 95814
(916) 445-8745

Hawaii

Ruth Larkin
Nursing Home Ombudsman
  Program
Commission on Aging
1149 Bethel Street, Rm. 311
Honolulu, Hawaii 96813
(808) 548-2593

Nevada

John R. Kimball

Nursing Home Ombudsman
  Program
Nevada Division on Aging
Department of Aging
Kinkead Bldg., Room 101
505 East King Street
Carson City, Nevada 89710

REGION X

Terry Duffin
Regional Liaison
Nursing Home Ombudsman
  Program
Office of Aging, DHEW Region X
Arcade Plaza Building
1321 Second Ave. — Mail Stop
  622
Seattle, Washington 98101
(206) 442-5341

Alaska

Nursing Home Ombudsman
  Program
Alaska Office on Aging
Pouch H OIC
Juneau, Alaska 99811
(907) 586-6153

Idaho

Arlene Warner, Director
Nursing Home Ombudsman
  Program
Idaho Office on Aging
Department of Special Services
State House
506 North 5th Street
Boise, Idaho 83707
(208) 384-3833

Oregon

Signa Livesay
Nursing Home Ombudsman
  Program
Human Resources Department
772 Commercial Street, S.E.
Salem, Oregon 97310
(503) 378-4728

Washington

Nursing Home Ombudsman
  Program
Washington Office on Aging
Department of Social and Health
  Services
Mail Stop 45-2
Olympia, Washington 98504
(206) 753-3393

DEPARTMENT OF HEALTH, EDUCATION, AND WELFARE

At the time of printing, HEW was being reorganized. It is therefore impossible to provide a list of specific individuals with responsibility for nursing homes. However, most letters or other inquiries addressed to the Honorable Joseph Califano, Secretary, Department of Health, Education, and Welfare, South Portal Building, Washington, D.C. 20201 will be directed to appropriate officers and receive immediate response. Specific problems which concern only *Medicare* may be addressed to Mr. Thomas Tierney, Director, Bureau of Health Insurance, 6401 Security Boulevard, Baltimore, Maryland 21235; telephone (301) 594-1234. Specific allegations of fraud in either program can be addressed to Mr. Tom Morris, Inspector General, HEW, Washington, D.C. 20201.

MAJOR SENIOR CITIZENS ORGANIZATIONS OR OTHER PROFESSIONAL GROUPS INTERESTED IN LONG TERM CARE

Virtually every major senior citizens organization has a strong interest in nursing home problems. The same can be said for many professional organizations. You may wish to contact these groups for assistance or for information. If you are a member of any of the following, you may want to encourage their efforts to improve the quality of nursing home care. If you need help you will find that many of these organizations are anxious to assist you in resolving complaints. Some such groups are beginning to compile inspection records and may be able to provide some guidance with respect to your choice of facilities.

National Council of Senior
Citizens
1511 K Street, N.W., Suite 520
Washington, D.C. 20005
(202) 783-6850

National Retired Teachers
Association — American
Association of Retired Persons
1909 K Street, N.W., Suite 621
Washington, D.C. 20006
(202) 872-4700

National Council on the Aging
1828 L Street, N.W., Suite 504
Washington, D.C. 20036
(202) 223-6250

National Farmers Union
1012 14th Street, N.W.
Washington, D.C. 20018
(202) 628-9774

Gerontological Society
#1 Dupont Circle — Suite 520
Washington, D.C. 20036
(202) 659-4698

National Association of Retired
Federal Employees
1533 New Hampshire Avenue,
N.W.
Washington, D.C. 20036
(202) 234-0832

National Council of Senior
Citizens Legal Research for the
Elderly
1511 K Street, N.W.
Washington, D.C. 20005
(202) 638-4351

National Caucus on the Black
Aged
1730 M Street, N.W., Suite 811
Washington, D.C. 20036
(202) 785-8766

Gray Panthers
3700 Chestnut Street
Philadelphia, Pennsylvania 19104
(215) 848-2038

National Senior Citizens Law
Center
1709 West 8th Street
Los Angeles, California 90017
(213) 483-3990

Federal Council on Aging
400 Sixth Street, S.W., Room 4022
Washington, D.C. 20201
(202) 245-0727

International Center for Social
Gerontology
425 13th Street, N.W., Room 350
Washington, D.C. 20004
(202) 393-0347

International Federation on
Ageing
1909 K Street, N.W., Room 350
Washington, D.C. 20004
(202) 872-4700

National Association of Area
Agencies on Aging
Central Bank Building, Room 350
Huntsville, Alabama 35801
(205) 533-3330

National Association of State
Units on Aging
State Office Building, 1123 Eutaw
Street
Baltimore, Maryland 21201
(301) 383-2100

Urban Elderly Coalition
c/o Office of Aging of New York
City
250 Broadway
New York, New York 10007
(212) 566-0154

American Jewish Congress
15 East 84th Street
New York, New York 10028
(212) 879-4500

California Rural Legal Assitance
942 Market Street
San Francisco, California 94102
(415) 989-3966

Congress of Senior Citizens
111 N.E. Second Avenue
Miami, Florida 33132
(305) 371-5678

Council of Elders, Inc.
1990 Columbus
Boston, Massachusetts 02119
(617) 442-1091

National Association of Social
  Workers
600 Southern Bldg.
15th & H Streets N.W.
Washington, D.C. 20005
(202) 628-6800

National League for Nursing
10 Columbus Circle
New York, New York 10019
(212) 582-1022

American Nurses Association
2420 Pershing Road
Kansas City, Missouri 64108
(816) 474-5720

American Medical Association
535 N. Dearborn St.
Chicago, Illinois 60610
(312) 751-6000

AFL-CIO
815 16th Street N.W.
Washington, D.C. 20006
(202) 637-5000

INDUSTRY ASSOCIATIONS

American Health Care Association (formerly American
  Nursing Home Association)
1200 15th Street N.W.
Washington, D.C. 20005
(202) 833-2050

American Association of Homes
  for the Aging
529 14th Street N.W.
Washington, D.C. 20005
(202) 347-2000

American Association of
  Consultant Pharmacists
2300 9th Street South, Suite 415
Alexandria, Virginia

National Council of Health Care
  Services
1200 15th Street N.W.
Washington, D.C. 20005
(202) 785-4754

American College of Nursing
  Home Administrators
Suite 409
8641 Colesville Road
Silver Spring, Maryland 20910
(301) 589-9070

NATIONAL CITIZENS COALITION FOR NURSING HOME REFORM

On June 10, 1975, representatives from 15 different citizens groups met in Washington, D.C. and established a national coalition to work for nursing home reform. The informal leader of the group is Elma Griesel formerly with Ralph Nader's retired Professional Action Group and the Gray Panther's Long-Term Care Action Project and presently with the National Paralegal Institute, 2000 P Street, N.W., Washington, D.C.; telephone (202) 872-0755. Also instrumental in establishing this important organization were Linda Horn of the Philadelphia Gray Panthers, Chuck Chomet, executive director of Citizens for Better Care, Detroit, Michigan and Patricia Powers formerly of the Citizens Monitoring Team, Davenport, Iowa.

Griesel and Horn have written *Nursing Homes: A Citizen's Action Guide*, published in paperback by Beacon Pres. It is a textbook telling how to set up your own consumer action group dedicated to nursing home improvement. The book is highly recommended. If you do not want to form your own group, you may wish to join or provide financial support for any of the following associated groups.

Gray Panthers
Long-Term Care Action Project
3700 Chestnut Street
Philadelphia, Pennsylvania 19104
(215) 382-3546

Citizens for Better Care
960 Jefferson Avenue E.
Detroit, Michigan 48207
(313) 963-0513

Citizens for the Improvement of
   Nursing Homes
9103 - 32nd Avenue N.E.
Seattle, Washington 98115
(206) 523-1211

Citizens for Better Nursing Home
   Care, Inc.
P.O. Box 90920
Milwaukee, Wisconsin 53202
(414) 224-0460

Denver Gray Panthers
1400 Lafayette
Denver, Colorado 80218
(303) 832-5618

Friends and Relatives of Nursing
   Home Patients
1765 East 26th
Eugene, Oregon 97403
(503) 343-7888

Minneapolis Age & Opportunity
   Center, Inc.
1801 Nicollet Ave. South
Minneapolis, Minnesota 55403
(612) 874-5525

National Consumers League
1785 Massachusetts Ave. N.W.
Washington, D.C. 20036
(202) 797-7600

New York Gray Panther Nursing
   Home Action Group
424 East 62nd Street
New York, New York, 10021
(212) 755-0876

Northwest Interfaith Movement
Greene St. at Westview
Philadelphia, Pennsylvania 19119
(215) 843-5600

Nursing Home Campaign
  Committee, Inc.
1547 Pratt Street
Philadelphia, Pennsylvania 19124
(215) 744-0882

Better Government Association
360 North Michigan Avenue
Chicago, Illinois 60601
(312) 641-1181

KEY CONGRESSIONAL CONTACTS

Honorable Frank Church,
  Chairman
Senate Committee on Aging
G-225 Dirksen Senate Building
Washington, D.C. 20510

Honorable Herman Talmadge,
  Chairman
Subcommittee on Health, Senate
  Finance Committee
Washington, D.C. 20510

Honorable Claude Pepper,
  Chairman
Select Committee on Aging
House of Representatives
Washington, D.C. 20515

Honorable Dan Rostenkowski,
  Chairman
Subcommittee on Health, House
  Ways and Means Committee
Washington, D.C. 20515

Honorable Paul Rogers,
  Chairman
Subcommittee on Health, House
  Interstate and Foreign
  Commerce Committee
Washington, D.C. 20515

Honorable Edward M. Kennedy,
  Chairman
Subcommittee on Health
Senate Committee on Human
  Resources
Washington, D.C. 20510

Chapter Notes

Introduction

1. *Vienna* (Georgia) *News*, 16 April 1970.

2. As quoted by William F. Buckley in his March 21, 1974, syndicated column.

Chapter 1

1. The welfare program which pays for nursing home care is called Medicaid. It is a grant-in-aid program administered by HEW wherein the federal government pays from 50 to 83 percent of the cost of nursing home care for state welfare recipients. About 60 percent of Medicaid funds are federal; the remainder are paid by the states. More than one-third of all Medicaid funds goes to pay for nursing home care; an additional 31 percent is paid to hospitals. In 1975, Medicaid paid over $5 billion out of its total $15 billion to nursing homes.

Medicaid pays for two levels of nursing home care, and facilities derive their names from the level of care they provide. Skilled nursing facilities (SNFs) provide skilled nursing care, the most intensive level of care, which is distinguished by the availability of licensed or professional nurses on duty 24 hours a day. Intermediate care facilities (ICFs) provide intermediate care which, as its name suggests, is more than board and room, but short of skilled nursing care. The typical ICF helps the patient perform activities necessary to his well being such as in eating, bathing, and taking medications. Skilled nursing care is presently available under both Medicare and Medicaid, while intermediate care is authorized only under Medicaid.

By contrast, Medicare is a 100 percent federal program whose benefits are available to all older Americans. Congress has authorized

100 days of nursing home care in a Medicare-approved facility for individuals over 65 or disabled meeting these conditions: they must have been hospitalized for three consecutive days; they must arrive at the nursing home within 14 days of their discharge from the hospital; and a physician must certify that they require skilled nursing in the extension of the kind of care for which they were hospitalized. The prior hospitalization requirements and a restrictive definition of those medical arts compensable under the definition of skilled nursing have limited the help Medicare provides to the infirm elderly. Out of the one million senior citizens in nursing homes, only 8,300 individuals on any given day have their care paid for by Medicare. Medicare pays for about two percent of the nation's nursing home bill.

Chapter 2

1. For more examples of documented nursing home abuses see Supporting Paper Number 1, in the series, "Nursing Home Care in the United States: Failure in Public Policy," a report of the Subcommittee on Long Term Care, Senate Committee on Aging, January 1975.

Still further examples can be found in the nation's case law. The *Nursing Home Law Manual*, published by the Health Law Center, Aspen Systems Corporation, is an excellent resource for any nursing home owner or administrator or any attorney with nursing home clients. For example, in the discussion of negligence by nursing home employees, the *Manual* cites such cases as *Hendricks v. Sanford*, 337 P.2d 974 (1959), in which the plaintiff sued a nursing home for failure to keep her bed clean. The patient eventually developed near-fatal bedsores. *Elliot v. Tempkins*, 299 N.Y.S.2d 857, 1969, involved a nurse who placed a paralyzed patient on a commode, tied him down, left him and served other patients lunch. The patient's cigarette dropped and his clothes caught fire. During the several minutes the aide was gone, the patient was unable to extinguish the fire and burned to death. *Ferguson v. Dr. McCarty's Rest Home*, 142 N.E.2d 337, 1957, concerned a paralyzed patient who suffered severe burns when her foot came into contact with a radiator by her bed. The patient screamed for an hour before the nurse could "pull herself together" and rescue her charge. *Smith v. Silver Spring-Wheaton Nursing Home*, 220 A.2d 574, 1966, involved an action against a nursing home which hired an allegedly insane practical nurse who beat up a patient. In another landmark case, *Dunahoo v. Brooks*, 128 So.2d 486, 1961, the court held a nursing home liable for injuries suffered by a 94-year-old woman patient who tripped and fell over a light cord lying loose on the floor by her bed.

Chapter 3

1. Edward S. Brady, *Drugs and the Elderly* (San Francisco: University of California, Ethel Percy Andrus Gerontology Center, 1973), p. 12.

Chapter 5

1. Obviously, an entire book could be written about this one aspect of the national nursing home problem. See for example, *Tender Loving Greed* by Mary Adelaide Mendelson.

2. Under existing laws it is impossible to tell who owns nursing homes. For example, the 1972 Governor's Commission on Nursing Home Problems, headed by Paul Kerschner, discovered just how ineffective federal laws were. After a great deal of effort, the commission threw up its hands in despair. Similar patterns were uncovered by the subcommittee in Minnesota, Florida, and Michigan. The Nader task force charged that this problem was national in scope and recommended that Congress find a better means of identifying nursing home owners. This recommendation adds further support to the need for penalties for noncompliance with the law.

The subcommittee learned that through informal connections, nursing home conglomerates, or "syndicates," may amount to nothing more or less than a conspiracy to exploit the sick and the aged. Researching land records in Chicago and correlating these with state nursing home disclosure lists, the Better Government Association of Chicago discovered interlocking ownership of about 25 percent of the nursing home beds in Chicago. The president of the BGA, John McEnerney, told the subcommittee:

> This issue first came to our attention when investigator Bill Recktenwald was working at the Park House Nursing Home. The administrator mentioned several other homes where Recktenwald could possibly work. When he inquired if they were owned by the same people, he was told, "They are all owned by a kind of syndicate."
>
> This "syndicate" theory has gathered strength and credence as our investigators have gone through the long list of nursing ownership supplied by Dr. Yoder to the Senate committee.

Four points should be made here:

a. A small group owns a great many nursing homes.
b. These homes and their operation are connected by virtue of

      interlocking ownership or interlocking directors.

c. These homes, as we saw at the last hearing, seem to be able to make extremely high profits while at the same time the homes or their representatives are constantly pushing the state for higher rates.

d. The same homes have been identified by the State and city as being continually in violation of State standards. Clearly, the homes owned by this syndicate are among the worst in the State. Their motive seems to be making money at the expense of the most under-represented minority group in our society. None of us, Mr. Chairman, condemns the profit motive which has helped build this country. However, we do vigorously condemn profiteering. The spectacle of those living the good life at the expense of the sick and dying certainly deserves the contempt of all good men everywhere.

Nor is this experience unique to Illinois. The Governor's Commission in Michigan looked at the nursing homes in Wayne County. The commission uncovered six interlocking networks which owned about a third of the 115 homes in Wayne County and about 40 percent of the 11,000 beds. In its September 1975 testimony, the Michigan Fraud Squad testified they had evidence of the involvement of organized crime in the ownership of nursing homes in that state. Similar suggestions and testimony have been received by the subcommittee concerning New Jersey, Illinois, New York, and Florida. The importance of a better federal law with respect to nursing home ownership is obvious.

3. No attempt has been made in this book to describe the complicated financial transactions which occur between the major nursing home chains. The full dimensions of less than arm's-length dealings, sale and lease-back operations, pyramiding mortgages, and the like are set forth in the subcommittee's report, "Profits and the Nursing Home: Incentives in Favor of Poor Care."

Chapter 6

1. *Patient Care Magazine*, March 30, 1972, p. 59.
2. Margaret Blenkner, monograph, "The Place of Nursing Homes Among Community Resources," 1965.

Chapter 7

1. Paraphrased from testimony before the Subcommittee on Long Term Care by Sharon Fujii, August 10, 1972.
2. Testimony before the Subcommittee on Long Term Care, August

10, 1972, "Trends in Long-Term Care," Part 20, Washington, D. C., pp. 2481-2496.

3. In 1975 and 1976 the Office of Civil Rights investigated 17 complaints of alleged racial discrimination in nursing homes.

Chapter 9

1. "Most of the problems in nursing homes can be traced to the profit motive, which is incompatible with social programs," according to a report issued in late February by the AFL-CIO. In order to correct the problems, *the labor union recommends that private, for-profit homes gradually be phased out* and replaced by religious, government, or other nonprofit homes.

The findings in *America's Nursing Homes: Profit in Human Misery* are based on a year-long investigation of 28 nursing homes undertaken by union volunteers and members of other community-based groups in 14 states. Inspection teams cited the failure of facilities to meet minimum fire safety standards, unsanitary conditions, abusive treatment of patients, and questionable financial practices as proof that many nursing home patients fail to receive even adequate care. Government reports of congressional and criminal investigations are cited in the report to bolster the findings of the AFL-CIO.

The AFL-CIO Executive Council is encouraging union members to continue monitoring nursing homes to improve conditions for patients. Copies of a statement by the Executive Council and the full report may be obtained from Leo Perlis, Department of Community Services, AFL-CIO, 815 16th Street, N.W., Washington, D.C. 20006.

2. Even when states report audits, they are, more often than not, desk audits, which involve checking arithmetic and little more, as opposed to in-depth field audits in which auditors verify each element of costs claimed for reimbursement.

Chapter 11

1. See Report of the Welfare Inspector General, State of New York, reprinted in hearings by the Subcommittee on Long Term Care, New York, New York, February 4, 1975.

Chapter 12

1. Ewald Busse, "Are MD's Wary of Treating the Aged Chronically Ill?" *Medical Journal*, March 27-28, 1965, p. 7.

2. *Patient Care Magazine*, March 30, 1973, p. 59.

3. Bernard A. Strotsky and Joan R. Dominick, "The Physician's Role in the Nursing Home and Retirement Home," *The Gerontologist*, Spring 1970, part II, p. 41.

4. *Minneapolis Morning Tribune*, 15 July 1969, p. 7.

Chapter 13

1. "Nursing Home Research Project — Report on Nurse Aides," Spring 1972, p. 3.

2. Quoted in subcommittee hearings, "Trends in Long-Term Care," St. Petersburg, Florida, January 9, 1970, p. 206.

Chapter 14

1. Quoted in subcommittee hearings, "Trends in Long-Term Care," Chicago, Illinois, September 14, 1971, pp. 1514-1515.

Chapter 15

1. *Federal Register*, October 3, 1974 (HEW regulations applying to nursing homes participating in the Medicare and Medicaid programs).

Index

107, 136, 243
See also House of Representatives,
U.S.; Senate, U.S.
Connecticut
nursing home profits study, 77-78,
81, 180
reimbursement system, 142, 143, 145
State Board of Charities, 5
Continuing education programs,
208-209, 239
See also Training
Cook County
Department of Health, 110
Department of Public Health, 156, 157
Department of Public Welfare, 129
Copeland bills, 109
Corporate ownership, 6, 76, 77,
82-85, 101
Cost of Living Council (CLC), 82,
140, 141
Cousin, Lionel Z., 46, 114,
171, 177, 191
Cruikshank, Nelson, 45, 128
Crystal Springs Rehabilitation
Center, 204
Curran, William J., 184
Cushman, Margaret, 23
Cyanide, 71

D

Dachowitz, Samuel, 163, 170
Dakota Nursing Home, 215-216
Dame, George, 26
Danielson, Gladys E., 179-180
Danube Nursing Home, 166, 167-168
Death certificates, 183-184
Deaths, 13, 20, 25, 26, 31, 32, 33,
90, 108, 112, 115, 119, 157, 180
decrease, 5
drug-related, 53, 56-57
epidemics, 13, 26, 182
fear of, 12-13
fire, 59, 60-62, 64, 65, 67,
68, 70, 110
nursing home rate, 10, 13
starvation, 28, 157
smoke inhalation, 69, 70
See also Suicide
De La Parte, Louis, 129
Dental care, 35
Depression, 4
Detier, Ida Mae, 191
Detroit Health Department, 27
Detroit News, 79
Di-Com Construction Company, 169

Digitalis, 43, 50, 180, 181, 182
Dignity
loss, 12, 36
maintenance, 202, 203, 224
Disabilities, 63, 142
fear of, 9
increase, 5, 40
Disclosure of ownership, 148
Discrimination, 118, 119, 121, 123,
124, 125, 126
Diuretics, 43, 50, 51, 182
Diuril, 51
Division of Senior Citizens in
Chicago, 109
Dock, William, 205
Dominick, Joan R., 182
Donnatal, 51
Douglass, Robert, 166
Drugs, 129
addiction, 51, 52, 53-54, 57
cost, 39, 40, 45, 53, 100
distribution, 17, 18, 30, 31,
41-42, 47, 57, 156, 227-228
error, 42-44, 57
experimental, 39, 54-57
interactions of, 48-51
laws, 18
number per patient, 40, 48
overuse, 113
prescription by phone, 41, 179,
181, 182
reactions, 48-56, 57
records, 30-31, 44
reimbursement, 99
storage, 30, 31
types used, 40, 44-45
See also Tranquilizers;
specific drugs
Duke University
Center for the Study of Aging, 177

E

Eckel, Emily, 23
Eckel, Fred M., 42
Edwards, Don, 125
Einhorn, Irving, 65, 68, 70
Elavil, 51
Elderly
drug expenses, 39, 53
drug reactions, 48-49
economic pressures, 9-10
facilities lacking for, 109-110, 113
fears of, 8-14
fire dangers for, 62-63

Hurd, T. Norman, 166, 167, 169
Hutton, William R., 46, 149
Hydrocarbons, 70
Hydrochloric acid, 70
Hydrofluoric acid, 70
Hydrogen chloride, 69
Hydrogen cyanide, 70
Hydrogen fluoride, 70
Hynes, Charles J., 91, 93,
    100, 129-130, 164, 169
Hypoglycemic drugs, 43

I

Idaho
    negligence investigation, 13
Idaho Statesman, 13
Identity
    loss of, 11, 12
Illinois
    Department of Health, 26, 32, 129, 153,
        155-156, 158, 159, 160
    Department of Mental Health and
        Developmental Disabilities, 109, 112
    Department of Public Health, 143
    reimbursement system, 142-143
    transfer of mental patients, 109-113
Illinois Extended Care Center, 112
Illinois land trust, 76
Illinois Legislative Investigating
    Commission, 112
Illinois State Psychiatric
    Association, 111
Illness
    fear of, 9
INA, 82
Incontinence, 18, 115, 142, 202, 203
Independence
    loss of, 12
Infectious diseases, 18, 31, 32, 182-183
Influenza epidemic, 26
In-home care. *See* Home
    health care
Injury
    deliberate, 11, 25-26
    negligent, 25, 27
Insanity
    fear of, 10-11
    See also Mentally impaired
Inspections, 17, 26, 30, 78, 110,
    112-113, 127, 133, 151
    advance notice, 154, 156
    cursory nature, 154-155
    fire, 71
    frequency, 153-154, 155

personal factors, 155
political interference, 158-159, 165
responsibility, 153
results ignored, 155-158
state health departments'
    attitude, 159-160
Inspectors
    training, 71
Institutional councils, 210
Institutionalization
    impact, 10, 11
Insulin, 43, 44, 181
Intermediate care facilities
    (ICF), 186, 220, 221
Internal Revenue Service, 85, 93
Investment returns, 74, 75, 76, 77,
    78, 80, 81, 84, 93
Iowa Soldiers' Home, 213-214

J

Jackson, Hobart, 121
Jackson, Jacquelyne, 121
Jewish Home and Hospital for the
    Aged, 208
Johns Hopkins University
    School of Medicine, 173
Johnson, Amos, 5, 103-104
Johnson, Gloria, 180
Johnson administration, 136
Joint Committee on the Accreditation
    of Hospitals, 67
Justice, Department of
    discrimination investigations, 125, 126

K

Kaas, Amram, 167
Kanamycin, 50
Kane, J.J., Hospital
    abuse of patients, 15-23
    beds, 15
    budget, 15
    deaths, 19
    discharges, 19
    investigation of, 15, 23-24
    patient stay, 19
Kansas
    nursing home investigation,
        30-31, 129
Kassel, Victor, 4, 176, 177,
    186-187, 191
Kastenbaum, Robert, 205
Katz, Allan, 44

About the Authors

Frank E. Moss was born in Holliday, Utah, on September 23, 1911. He graduated from Utah public schools and received his B.A. in 1933 from the University of Utah. In 1937, he received his J.D. from George Washington University. He spent the next two years as an attorney with the Securities and Exchange Commission and was elected Salt Lake County judge in 1940—an office to which he was re-elected in 1945. He served four years as a judge advocate in the European Theater during World War II and is a retired colonel of the United States Air Force Reserve. He was elected Salt Lake County Attorney in 1950 and re-elected in 1954. He twice was elected president of the National District Attorneys Association. He was elected to the United States Senate where he served three terms from 1959 through 1976. As chairman of the Consumer Subcommittee on the Senate Commerce Committee, he established himself as the Senate's foremost champion of the consumer. He is an acknowledged expert on energy, water, and land management. He served as chairman of the Senate Aeronautics and Space Committee. He also became the Senate's leading expert on aging and long term care. Since 1963, he has conducted some 60 hearings dealing with one or more aspects of long term care.

Val J. Halamandaris was born in Price, Utah, on September 25, 1942. He was educated in Utah public schools and received his B.A. from George Washington University in 1966. In 1969 he received his J.D. from Catholic University School of Law and began work with the Senate Special Committee on Aging, where he currently holds the post of associate counsel. As of December 1976, he had personally set up 49 hearings, written 15 reports and drafted over 100 bills. He directed all the activities of the Subcommittee on Long Term Care, including investigations into nursing home abuses and other related aspects of Medicare and Medicaid fraud and abuse. He is an expert in the fields of aging, health, and long term care and has made numerous appearances on national television shows, including "The David Susskind Show" and CBS "Sixty Minutes." He is a member of the bar of the Supreme Court of the United States and the United States Court of Appeals for the District of Columbia. He is a member of the American Bar Association, the D.C. Bar Association, and the Health Lawyers Association. He also serves on the National Capital Medical Foundation Long Term Care Committee, a Washington, D.C. Professional Standards Review Organization. His writings have appeared in various periodicals. An amateur photographer, his works have appeared in such publications as *Newsweek*, the *New York Times* and the *Washington Post*.